Medical Ophthalmology
Examinations

J. Cohen

51   18 25 27
101   61 127 76
167

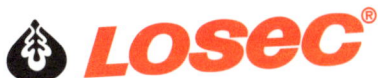

Medical Ophthalmology for Postgraduate Examinations

R.J. Morris BSc MRCP FRCS FCOphth
Senior Registrar in Ophthalmology, Moorfields Eye Hospital,
London, UK

J.E. MacSweeney BSc MRCP
Registrar in Radiology, Royal Postgraduate Medical School, Hammersmith
Hospital, London; formerly Registrar in Neurology and Medical
Ophthalmology, St Thomas' Hospital, London, UK

Foreword by
Michael D. Sanders FRCP FRCS FCOphth
Consultant Ophthalmologist, National Hospital for Nervous Diseases,
London and St Thomas' Hospital, London, UK

Churchill Livingstone
EDINBURGH LONDON MELBOURNE NEW YORK AND TOKYO
1991

CHURCHILL LIVINGSTONE
Medical Division of Longman Group UK Limited

Distributed in the United States of America by
Churchill Livingstone Inc., 1560 Broadway, New York,
N.Y. 10036, and by associated companies, branches
and representatives throughout the world.

First published 1991

ISBN 0-443-04049-4

British Library Cataloguing in Publication Data
Morris, R. J.
    Medical ophthalmology for postgraduate examinations.
    1. Ophthalmology
    I. Title II. MacSweeney, J. E.
    617.7

Library of Congress Cataloging in Publication Data.
Morris, R. J. (Robert John), FCOphth
    Medical ophthalmology for postgraduate examinations/
    R. J. Morris, J. E. MacSweeney; foreword by Michael D. Sanders.
    p. cm.
    ISBN 0–443–04049–4
    1. Ophthalmology—Examinations, questions, etc.
    I. MacSweeney, J. E. (Josephine Emir) II. Title.
    [DNLM: 1. Eye Diseases—examination questions.
    WW 18 M877m]
    RE49.M67 1991
    617.7′ 0076–dc20
    DNLM/DLC
    for Library of Congress

Produced by Longman Group (FE) Ltd
Printed in Hong Kong

Foreword

This book by an ophthalmologist and a physician contains questions presenting many of the common and important problems of medical ophthalmology. The large number of wide-ranging and well-illustrated cases, each with a concise discussion, makes this a very worthy educational supplement.

M.D.S.

Acknowledgements

We would like to thank Mr Michael Sanders, who has stimulated our interest in the subjects of medical and neurophthalmology and who provided valuable advice in the preparation of this text. The majority of the illustrations in this book have been provided by him and Dr Ross Russell from the departments of medical photography at St Thomas' Hospital and the National Hospital for Nervous Diseases. Ms N Poplar gave advice in the preparation of these slides. We are also grateful to other colleagues who allowed us to use their photographs; they include Mr P Rosen (Questions 11, 29, 78, 88, 93), Mr J Elston (Questions 9, 24, 36), Mr J R O Collin (Questions 14, 52, 63, 94), Dr T W Evans (Questions 1, 2, 57), Dr H L C Beynon (Questions 65, 86), Professor D Allison and Dr Adams (Questions 4, 8, 20), Mr D Taylor (Questions 56, 77), Mr C Migdal (Questions 49, 74), Dr G F Judisch (Question 50), Dr J Ruben (Question 70), Dr J. Nerad (Questions 24, 45, 66, 69), Ms C Ainslie (Questions 20, 44, 54, 73, 80, 82, 96) and Ms N Poplar (Questions 91, 98).

Preface

Medical ophthalmology is becoming increasingly recognised as a subject relevant to both surgical and medical disciplines. Consequently it forms an important part of both the written and clinical MRCP(UK) Part II examination, the FRCS examination and the FCOphth examination. Our aim in writing this book was to help the examination candidate prepare for both the written and oral parts of the examination, but it is not designed to be a comprehensive review of the subject.

The book contains 100 questions which cover those topics which are commonly asked in examinations. They are designed to test the candidate's ability not only to diagnose the ocular complaint and to suggest further investigations and treatment, but also to test their understanding of associated medical conditions. Each question is displayed on a right-hand page with its answer overleaf, accompanied by an explanation and further relevant information.

We hope that this book will ease the burden of examination candidates and also be useful to others interested in the subject.

London   R.J.M.
1991   J.E.MacS.

Question 1

1. What abnormality is present:
   (a) on the retina?
   (b) on the CT scan?
2. What is the diagnosis?

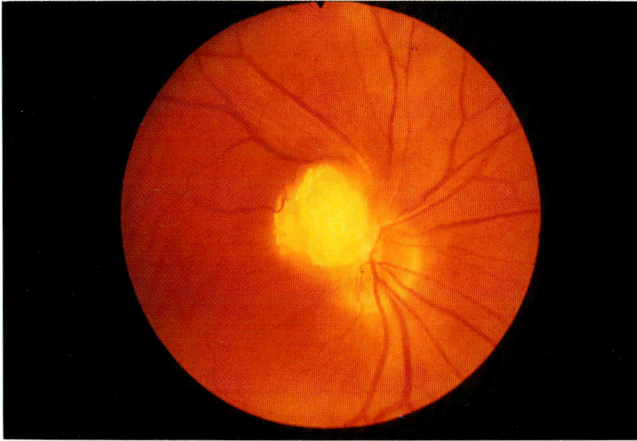

A

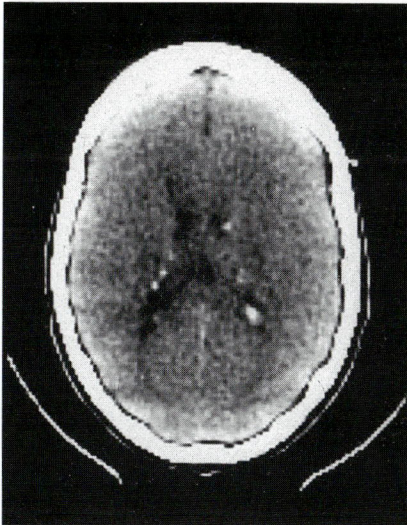

B

Answer to question 1

1. (a) Retinal phakoma (astrocytoma).
   (b) Tubers, calcified masses around the lateral ventricles.
2. Tuberous sclerosis (Bournville's disease, epiloia).

Tuberous sclerosis is an autosomal dominant condition characterised by mental retardation, epilepsy and adenoma sebaceum. Isolated cases are frequent, probably the result of spontaneous mutations. Cutaneous lesions consist of hypomelanotic macules developing in infancy and readily seen under ultraviolet light (Wood's lamp). Later in life adenoma sebaceum develop, as does the classical 'sharkskin' or shagreen patch on the lower back. Subungual fibromas may also be seen. Cerebral changes give rise to mental retardation and behavioural disorders in childhood. Epilepsy may occur even in patients with normal intelligence. Tuberous masses consisting of proliferative astrocytes distort and broaden the gyri and may calcify. They are found throughout the brain and extend into the ependymomas of the lateral ventricles and give rise to a characteristic 'candle guttering' radiological appearance. Malignant change may occur in these lesions. Retinal phakomas are discrete white gliomatous tumours of the retina, usually situated near the optic nerve head. They occur in 50% of patients and are bilateral in 15%.

Question 2

A 14-year-old boy presented with this rash one week after treatment for an upper respiratory tract infection.

1. What is the diagnosis?
2. Name two causes.
3. What are the ocular manifestations in the acute stage?

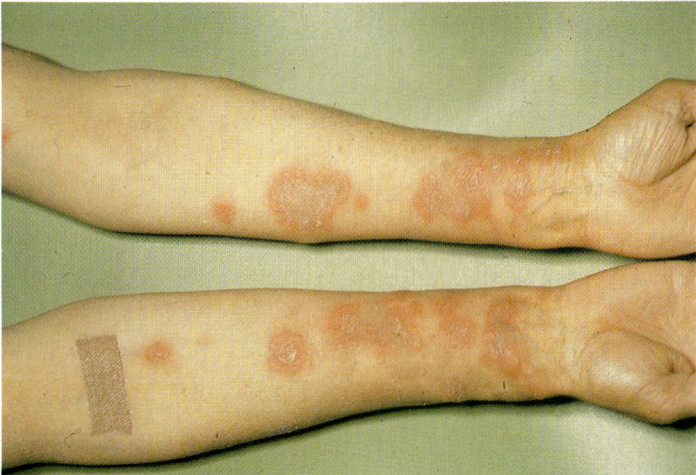

Answer to question 2

1. Erythema multiforme (Stevens–Johnson syndrome).
2. (a) Infections: most commonly herpes simplex and *Mycoplasma pneumoniae.*
  (b) Drugs: sulphonamides, penicillin and barbiturates.
  (c) Other causes: leukaemia, radiotherapy, SLE.
3. Conjunctival inflammation varies in severity from mild hyperaemia to marked bullous formation and ulceration. Secondary infection may follow ulceration.

Erythema multiforme is an acute hypersensitivity reaction (type III) in which vasculitis is precipitated by circulating immune complexes. It is seen most frequently in young males and has an acute onset with fever, malaise, sore throat, cough and arthralgia. The rash has a characteristic distribution involving the flexor surfaces of the arms and legs, the palms and back of the hands, spreading to involve the trunk. The lesions begin as erythematous macules often with a pale centre, may ulcerate and are surrounded by a circle of bright erythema (target lesion). They enlarge and tend to blister but heal without scarring.

The severe form of the disease with mucous membrane involvement leading to oral, ocular and genital ulceration, associated with fever and toxaemia, is known as Stevens–Johnson syndrome. Patients may develop dehydration, secondary infection, renal and pulmonary involvement. The conjunctival ulcerative changes heal with subepithelial fibrosis which may involve the lacrimal ductules to produce a dry eye. Symblepharon formation frequently follows ocular involvement and cicatricial entropion together with metaplastic lashes is seen in severe cases. These changes may lead to corneal vascularisation and opacification. Treatment with intensive topical steroids during the acute phase suppresses the inflammation and may reduce the extent of the cicatricial sequelae.

Question 3

What is the differential diagnosis?

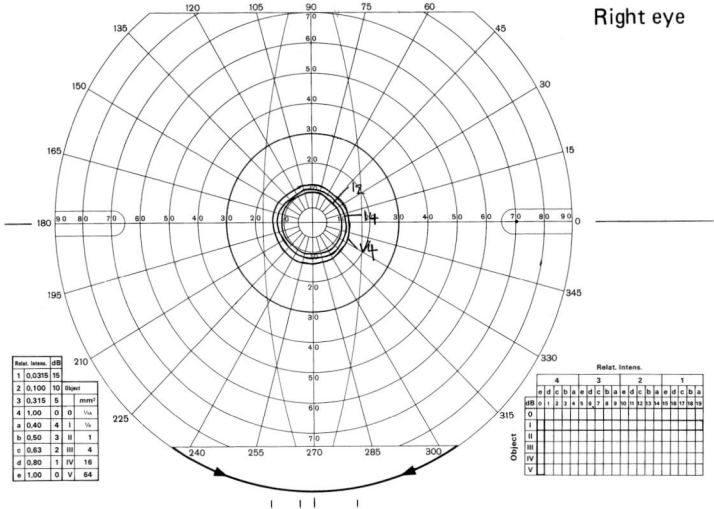

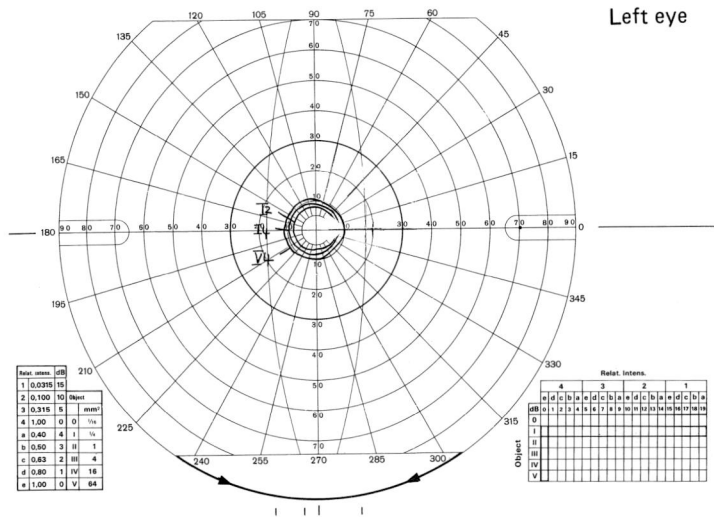

Right eye

Left eye

Answer to question 3

(a) Retinitis pigmentosa.
(b) End-stage glaucoma.
(c) Bilateral occipital lobe infarction with macular sparing.
(d) Extensive chorioretinitis.
(e) Chronic papilloedema.
(f) Hysteria.

When examining patients with organic visual field constriction the size of the field increases with testing distance and there is a separation between the isoptres on perimetry. The underlying cause can usually be identified by careful examination of the fundus. The visual field size does not change with different testing distances in the case of a functional constriction resulting in a tubular field pattern. In addition, on perimetry all isoptres tend to fall close to, or cross, each other, and some patients will show a spiral visual field, i.e. one that gradually expands as the target is moved circumferentially.

The patient can often be manipulated to produce the field desired by his examiner.

Question 4

This is the MRI scan of a 22-year-old woman who presented with blurring of vision in the right eye.

1. What abnormality is shown?
2. What is the likely cause for her visual disturbance?
3. What is the likely underlying diagnosis?

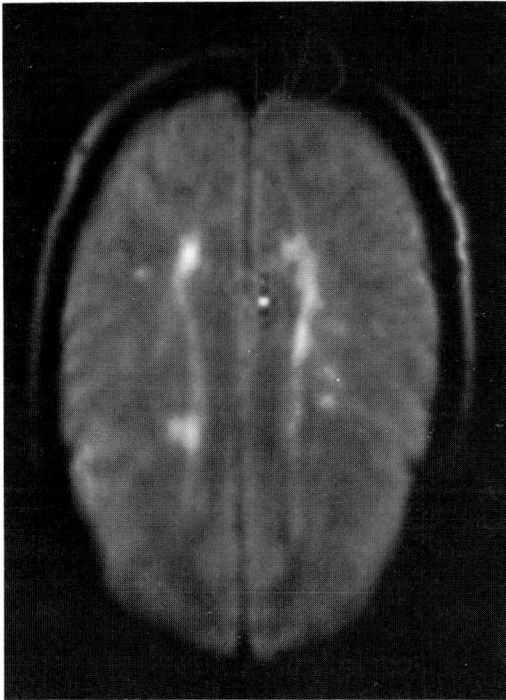

Answer to question 4

1. Multiple periventricular lucencies.
2. Optic neuritis.
3. Multiple sclerosis.

About 25% of all patients who develop multiple sclerosis (MS) present with an episode of optic neuritis. Magnetic resonance imaging is highly sensitive in detecting central nervous system white matter lesions in patients with MS. Optic nerve lesions may be visualised using a STIR sequence, and a T_2 weighted spin echo scan of the brain shows extensive high signal areas in the periventricular regions. These findings are not, however, specific for MS and may also be seen in other conditions such as cerebrovascular disease and cerebral infection. Multifocal white matter lesions are seen in over 90% of patients with clinically definite MS and 50–70% of adults with clinically isolated optic neuritis. In MS both oedema in acute lesions and gliosis in chronic disease are thought to explain the abnormal MRI signals. Approximately 75% of patients will have developed MS within 15 years of an acute attack of optic neuritis and the risk is higher in women than men; the risk does not decline after the first few years and the proportion of patients developing the disease steadily increases.

Question 5

What is the diagnosis?

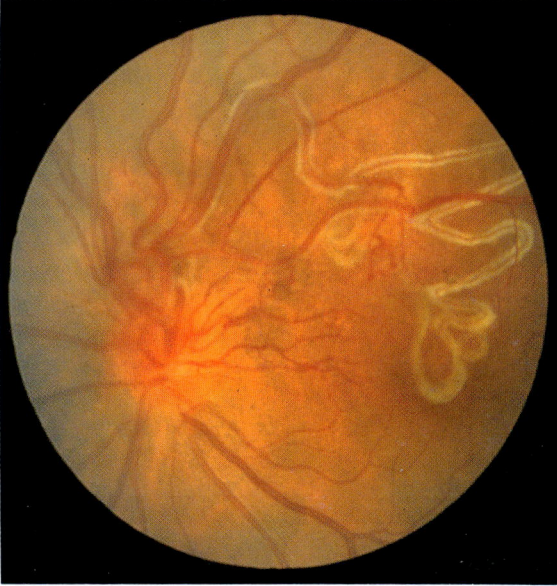

Answer to question 5

Arterio-venous malformation of the retinal vessels (racemose haemangioma).

Despite the dramatic appearance of large fundal arteriovenous malformations the lesions are usually asymptomatic. Visual acuity is affected only if the macula is involved. Frank vitreous haemorrhage is very rare. Wyburn-Mason syndrome is the association of retinal and mid-brain arteriovenous malformations.

Question 6

This patient returned to her general practitioner two days after being treated for an irritable left eye.

What is the diagnosis?

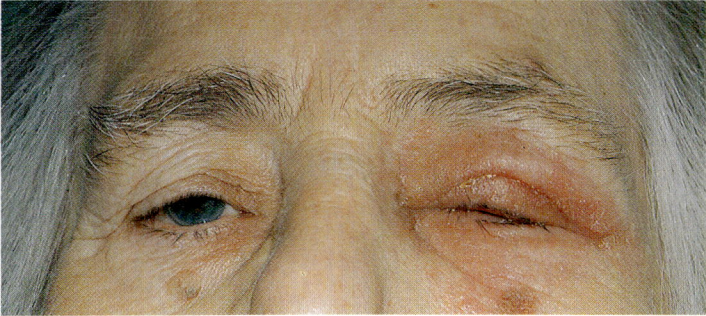

Answer to question 6

Contact dermatitis.

The slide shows the typical appearance of contact dermatitis with swelling of the lids, hyperaemia and crusting which in this patient was the result of a chloramphenicol allergy. Many eyedrops and ointments have the potential to cause allergic reactions, particularly those containing antibiotics. A similar but usually less severe picture may result from use of makeup and aerosol products or exposure to dust, chemicals and volatile solvents at work. Patch testing may help identify the allergenic chemical. The nature of the disorder should be explained to patients and in some cases a mild topical steroid may help in the short term.

Question 7

This is a slit-lamp photograph of a 50-year-old Jamaican woman who presented with blurred vision.

1. What is the abnormality shown?
2. What is the likely underlying systemic disease?

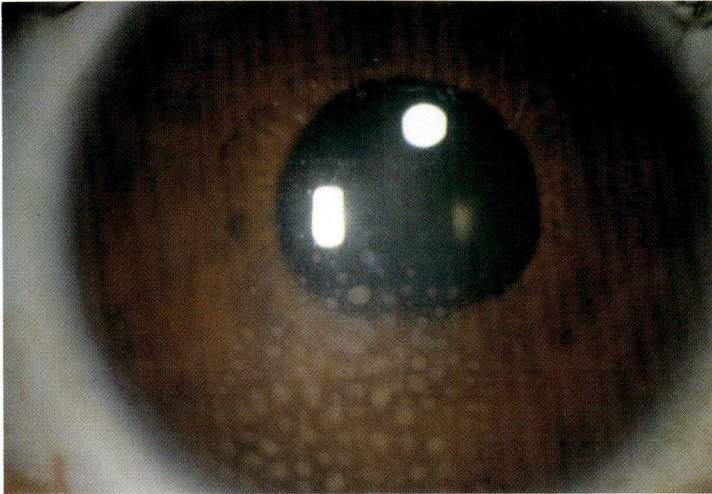

Answer to question 7

1. Keratic precipitates (mutton fat).
2. Sarcoidosis.

Twenty-five per cent of patients with sarcoidosis have ocular involvement at some stage and uveitis is the most common manifestation of ocular sarcoidosis. Anterior uveitis may be acute or chronic; the acute form typically affects young patients and may be associated with erythema nodosum and hilar lymphadenopathy; the chronic form is usually seen in older patients and may be complicated by band keratopathy, cataract and glaucoma. Posterior uveitis and retinal vasculitis may occur in the absence of anterior uveitis in some patients and candle wax exudates due to focal periphlebitis are typical; rarely neovascularisation may occur.

Sarcoid granulomas may affect the eyelids and conjunctiva; lacrimal gland infiltration is often seen, particularly in black Americans. Choroidal lesions vary in size from small granulomas to large masses and heal leaving atrophic scars. The optic disc may be swollen as a result of local oedema, granulomatous infiltration or papilloedema from raised intracranial pressure in patients with neurosarcoidosis. Facial nerve and other cranial nerve palsies may also be seen in this group of patients.

Question 8

1. What abnormalities are shown?
2. What three important tests would you perform to further assess this patient?
3. What is the most likely diagnosis?

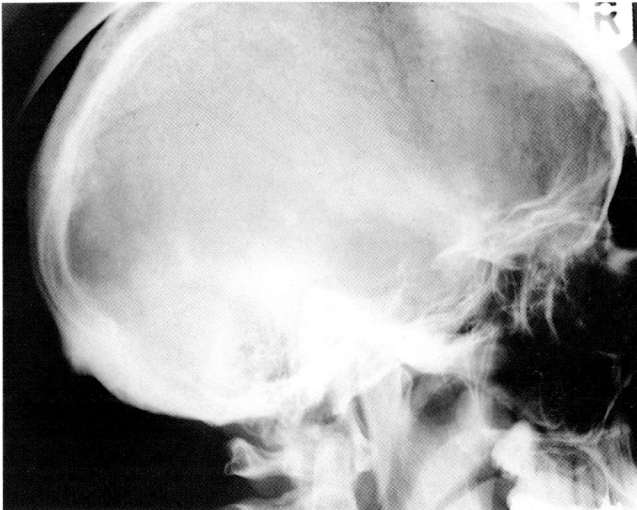

Answer to question 8

1. Enlargement of the pituitary fossa with erosion of the clinoid processes.
2. (a) CT scan of the head.
   (b) Pituitary function tests.
   (c) Visual fields.
3. A large pituitary tumour.

An enlarged pituitary fossa with erosion of the fossa floor is usually due to a pituitary tumour although CT scan occasionally reveals an empty fossa. The latter may occur secondary to infarction of the tumour at an earlier date, or, in the presence of craniostenosis, it may be due to chronically raised intracranial pressure and 'thumb printing' of the cranial vault may be seen on skull X-ray.

Question 9

1. What is:
   (a) the abnormality shown?
   (b) the diagnosis?
2. Name one ocular complication.
3. Name two neurological complications.
4. What abnormality would you expect to see on skull X-ray?

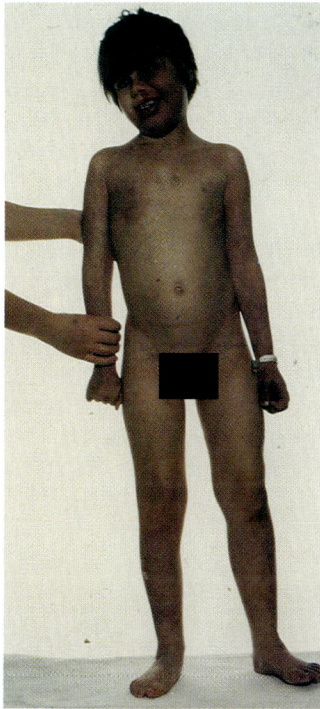

Answer to question 9

1. (a) Port wine vascular naevus in the territory of the fifth cranial nerve.
   (b) Sturge–Weber syndrome.
2. (a) Congenital glaucoma (buphthalmos).
   (b) Choroidal haemangioma — diffuse or localised.
   (c) Dilatation of conjunctival and episcleral vessels.
   (d) Heterochromia of the iris.
3. (a) Contralateral focal epilepsy (Jacksonian).
   (b) Contralateral spastic hemiparesis.
   (c) Contralateral hemisensory deficit.
   (d) Mental deficiency.
4. 'Tramline' calcification outlining convolutions of the parieto-occipital cerebral cortex.

Fifty per cent of patients have glaucoma on the side of the lesion, which is seen most frequently when the angioma affects the upper lid. It usually develops during childhood but may be seen in infancy. Cerebral involvement is due to angiomatous malformation of the leptomeninges of the parieto-occipital cortex and is associated strongly with involvement and of the second division of the fifth cranial nerve.

Question 10

1. Name three abnormalities shown on this fundus photograph.
2. What is the diagnosis?

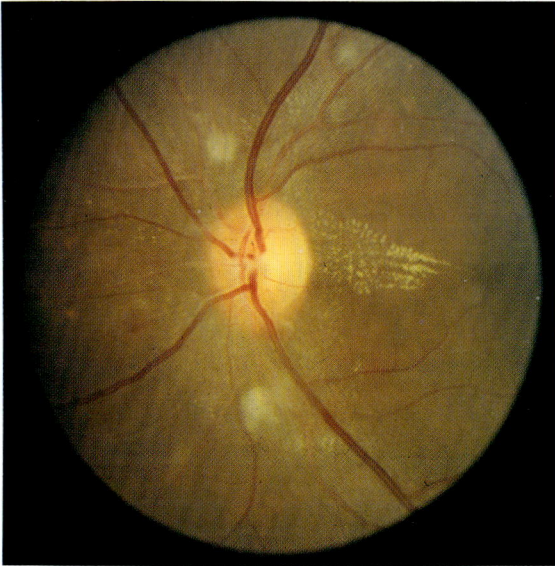

Answer to question 10

1. Cotton wool spots, retinal haemorrhages, arteriovenous nipping, hard exudates in the configuration of a macular star.
2. Hypertensive retinopathy.

Systemic hypertension produces changes in the choroidal, retinal and optic disc circulation. The extent of these changes depends on the age of the patient and the severity and duration of the hypertension. The early changes of hypertension are impossible to differentiate from the changes of arteriolosclerotic retinopathy. Hypertensive retinopathy may be classified into four grades (Wagener and Keith), with the five-year survival falling from 79% in group 1 to 1% in group 4.

Grade 1: Mild generalised arteriolar attenuation producing changes in the reflexes of the arteriolar wall (silver wiring and copper wiring).

Grade 2: Focal arteriolar attenuation including constriction of retinal arteries and arteriovenous nipping.

Grade 3: Cotton wool spots, hard exudates and retinal haemorrhages most commonly flame-shaped (nerve fibre layer).

Grade 4: Consists of all grade 3 changes plus disc swelling.

Patients with acute and severe hypertension often have florid grade 3 and 4 changes with few arteriolar changes which tend to indicate longstanding disease.

Question 11

This is a slit-lamp photograph of an eye of a young man with no history of ocular disease.

1. What is the most likely diagnosis?
2. List three ocular features of this condition.
3. What is the main cause of death?
4. What is the differential diagnosis?

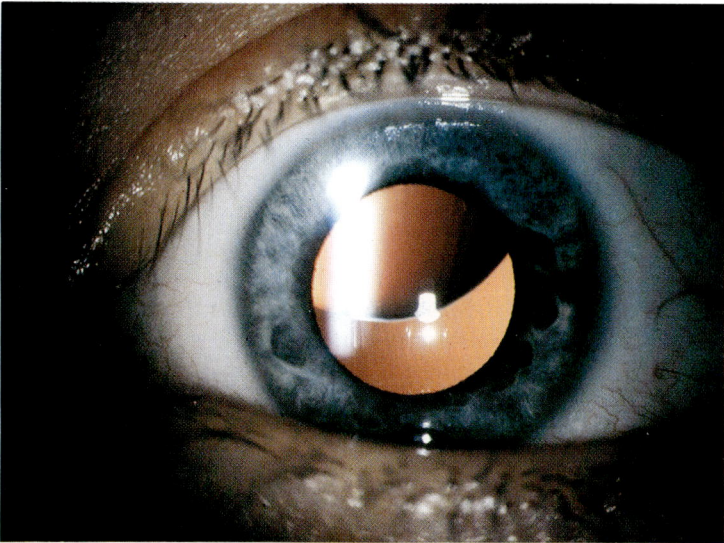

Answer to question 11

1. Marfan's syndrome.
2. (a) Upward subluxation of the lens (occurs in 80% of cases and is usually bilateral, symmetrical and non-progressive).
   (b) Glaucoma.
   (c) Myopia.
   (d) Retinal detachment.
3. Aortic dissection due to cystic medial necrosis of the aorta.
4. Homocystinuria.

Marfan's syndrome is a dominantly inherited disease characterised by widespread abnormalities of the connective tissue. The diagnosis is based on clinical findings, which in addition to the ocular features include tall stature with an armspan greater than height, arachnodactyly, high arched palate, scoliosis, and weakness of joint capsules, ligaments and tendons resulting in recurrent dislocation of joints and herniae. The commonest cardiovascular abnormalities described are aortic incompetence, dissecting aneurysms and mitral valve prolapse. The main differential diagnosis is homocystinuria in which the skeletal features are similar but the patients are mentally retarded and have light-coloured hair and no evidence of aortic incompetence. They do, however, have abnormalities of platelet function which may lead to life-threatening thromboses, particularly following general anaesthetics. Most important in the clinical differentiation is that the lens dislocates downwards in homocystinuria.

Question 12

1. What is the diagnosis?
2. What is the main complication?
3. List four other features of this disorder.

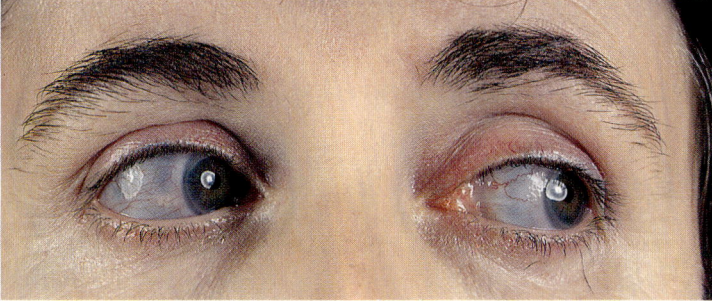

Answer to question 12

1. Osteogenesis imperfecta.
2. Excessive fragility of bones.
3. (a) Deafness (due to otosclerosis).
   (b) Hypermobility of joints.
   (c) Dentinogenesis imperfecta due to defective dentine.
   (d) Thin skin.
   (e) Cardiac valve lesions: aortic incompetence and redundant mitral valve.

Osteogenesis imperfecta comprises a group of inherited disorders in which abnormal synthesis of collagen is the common factor, the severity of which may vary from mild to very severe. Survivors in the latter group are severely deformed with a short bowed legs, kyphoscoliosis and a misshapen skull. A hyperplastic callus may develop which clinically may mimic a sarcoma.

Medical treatment is largely ineffective, and orthopaedic procedures are directed towards stabilising of fractures and correction of skeletal deformities.

Question 13

This child was asymptomatic.

What is the diagnosis?

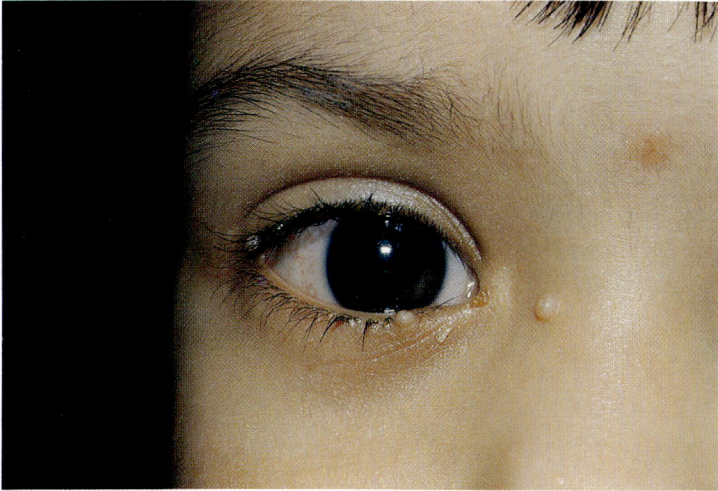

Answer to question 13

Molluscum contagiosum.

Molluscum contagiosum is a viral skin infection which is usually seen in children and most commonly affects the skin of the face and eyelids. The skin lesions may be single or multiple with a characteristic appearance. Typically they are elevated, dome-shaped and pearly white in colour with umbilicated centres. If the lesions are present at or near the lid margin the virus particles may be shed into the conjunctival sac and produce a secondary follicular conjunctivitis. The lesions disappear spontaneously in 6–9 months but if associated with a conjunctivitis should be removed.

Question 14

What is the diagnosis?

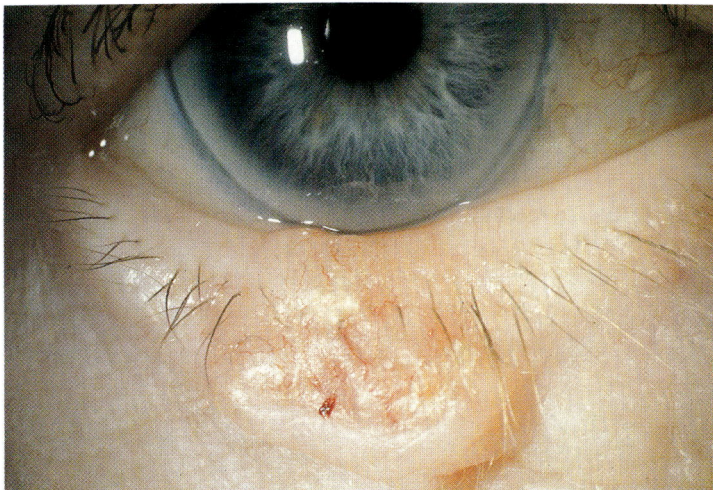

Answer to question 14

Basal cell carcinoma of the eyelid.

Basal cell carcinoma is the commonest malignant tumour of the eyelid and is seen most frequently on the lower lid and medial canthus. The classic appearance is of a central ulcer with a raised pearly margin with fine blood vessels on its surface. Basal cell carcinomas enlarge slowly and are locally invasive but do not metastasise. They may be treated by either surgery, cryotherapy or radiotherapy. Other less common eyelid tumours include squamous cell carcinomas, malignant melanomas and meibomian gland carcinomas.

Question 15

This 40-year-old woman has recurrent episodes of facial swelling.

1. What is the diagnosis?
2. Name two other clinical features.
3. What investigations would you perform to confirm the diagnosis?

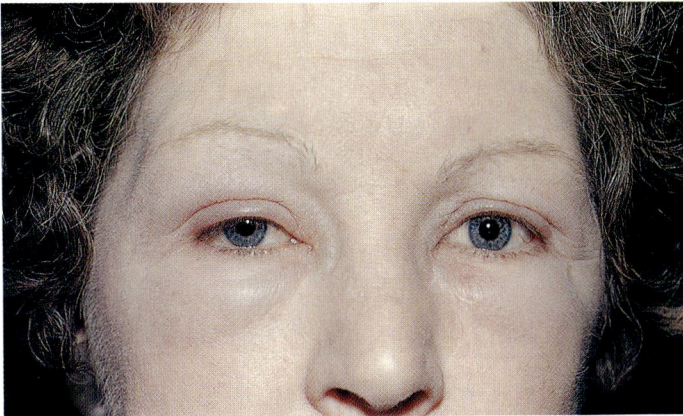

Answer to question 15

1. Angioedema.
2. (a) Recurrent colic from bowel involvement.
   (b) Urticarial whealing.
   (c) Oedema of the upper respiratory tract causing stridor.
3. Reduced serum C1 esterase inhibitor levels.

Angioedema is an autosomal dominant condition. It should be suspected in patients with a family history or those with previous episodes of prolonged swelling following minor trauma. Diagnosis is confirmed by the presence of low levels of serum neuroaminoglycoprotein C1 esterase inhibitor. Death is often the result of upper respiratory tract oedema.

Prophylaxis includes avoidance of trauma, especially in the region of the head and neck, and Danazol® 200 mg once daily, or during attacks Danazol® 400 mg per day. Fresh plasma containing C1 esterase may be given prior to surgical procedures or during an attack.

Question 16

This 24-year-old Turkish male with a history of recurrent oral and genital ulceration presented with reduced vision in his right eye.

1. What is the diagnosis?
2. Name two other clinical features of the disease.

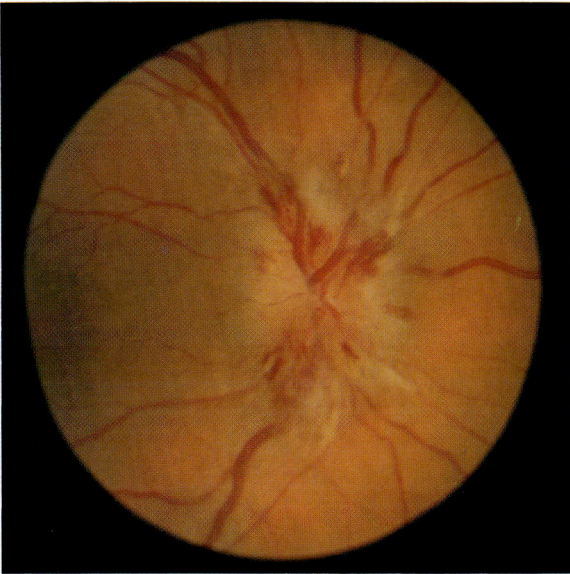

Answer to question 16

1. Behçet's disease.
2. (a) Thrombophlebitis leading to occlusion of superficial veins and occasionally the superior and inferior vena cava.
   (b) Arthritis, most commonly affecting the knees.
   (c) Skin rashes: erythema nodosum, vesiculopapular eruptions and pustules, particularly on the feet and trunk.
   (d) Meningoencephalitis.
   (e) Gastrointestinal, cardiovascular and renal involvement may also occur.

The diagnosis of Behçet's disease is based on the clinical triad of recurrent oral ulceration, genital ulceration and uveitis. The disease is seen most frequently in Mediterranean and Middle Eastern males but is being increasingly recognised in Caucasians. The basic pathology is an obliterative vasculitis predominantly affecting veins.

Ocular involvement occurs in 70% of cases and is related to HLA-B5. Severe uveitis is common with iritis often occurring in the presence of a white eye. Branch vein occlusion in the presence of severe uveitis is characteristic of the disease; other retinal signs include diffuse retinal oedema, optic disc oedema and in severe disease massive retinal exudation.

The visual prognosis before the advent of immunosuppresive therapy was extremely poor with 70% of patients going blind in both eyes. Although some patients respond to high-dose corticosteroid therapy alone, in others azathioprine or chlorambucil may have to be used in addition.

Question 17

This 34-year-old woman is attempting to look to her left. She presented with an acute onset of dizziness and horizontal diplopia. Two years ago she had an episode of paraesthesia in the right arm and leg lasting two weeks and on examination she had pyramidal signs in the right leg.

1. What is the abnormality of ocular movement?
2. What are the features of this abnormality?
3. What is the clinical diagnosis?

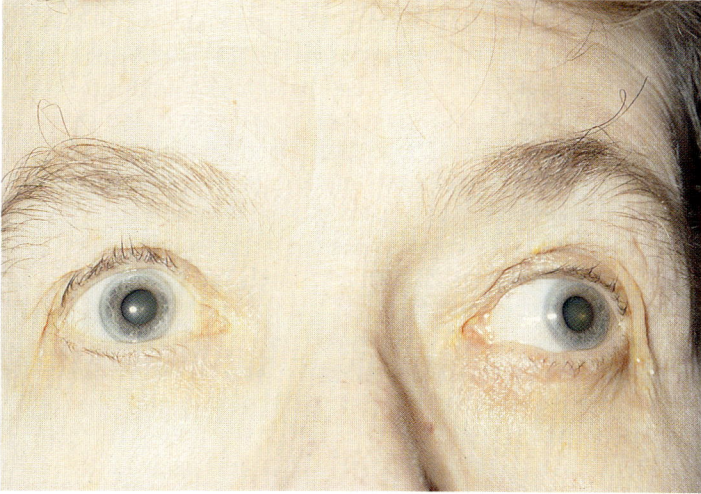

Answer to question 17

1. Internuclear ophthalmoplegia.
2. Reduced adduction of the eye on the affected side with slow saccades and nystagmus in the abducting eye.
3. Multiple sclerosis.

An internuclear ophthalmoplegia is caused by a lesion of the medial longitudinal fasciculus (MLF) on the same side. The eyes are often straight in the primary position, convergence may be normal or impaired and vertical nystagmus is frequently seen on upgaze. Partial lesions of the MLF may lead to a lag of the adducting eye when compared to the abducting eye; this is best seen when saccadic movements are carried out and the slowness of the adducting eye can be seen. Using the optokinetic drum the adducting eye on the side of the lesion will lag during the quick phase (the refixation saccade) of optokinetic nystagmus when compared to the abducting eye.

Bilateral internuclear ophthalmoplegia is most frequently due to multiple sclerosis. Unilateral lesions may be due to demyelination, vascular disease and rarely an intrinsic or extra-axial brainstem tumour.

An internuclear ophthalmoplegia can be mimicked by myasthenia gravis, thyroid eye disease and squint surgery.

It is important look for features in the history and examination which may differentiate between these conditions.

Question 18

This 14-year-old girl presented with diplopia and progressive swelling of the upper lid three weeks after an upper respiratory tract infection.

1. What is the likely diagnosis?
2. What two investigations should be performed?

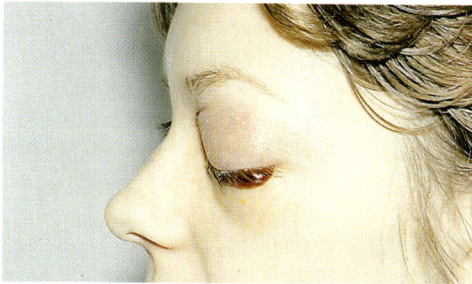

Answer to question 18

1. Orbital cellulitis.
2. Sinus and orbital X-rays and blood cultures (and cultures from nasopharynx and sinuses).

Orbital cellulitis is an uncommon disease, seen mainly in children, which in the preantibiotic era was associated with a mortality of 20–50% and blindness in 20–55% of survivors. Orbital infections most commonly arise from bacterial sinusitis; other predisposing factors include dental abscesses, orbital or strabismus surgery, local suppuration of the skin, orbital fractures and intraorbital foreign bodies.

Preseptal cellulitis presents with diffuse swelling of the upper lid. Signs of post-septal involvement include chemosis, proptosis, restricted ocular motility, pain on ocular movement, and signs of optic nerve dysfunction. The organisms most commonly responsible include *Haemophilus influenzae* (particularly in children under four years), *Streptococcus pneumoniae, Streptococcus pyogenes, Staphylococcus aureus* and anaerobic bacteria. Treatment with appropriate parenteral antibiotics should be commenced as soon as specimens for bacterial culture have been taken. In patients not responding to antibiotic therapy CT scans (or MRI scans) of the orbit should be performed. Surgery is indicated in patients with subperiosteal or orbital abscesses, decreasing vision and orbital foreign bodies.

Complications include cavernous sinus thrombosis, subdural empyema, cerebral abscess, meningitis, blindness and permanent restriction of ocular motility.

Question 19

A 45-year-old woman presented with deterioration of vision in the right eye which she noticed when covering the left eye. On examination her visual acuity was 6/60 R and 6/6 L, she had absent colour vision in the right eye with a right relative afferent pupillary defect and slight pallor of the right optic disc. Her visual fields are shown below.

1. What is the site of the pathology?
2. What is the most likely underlying pathology?
3. Name two important investigations.

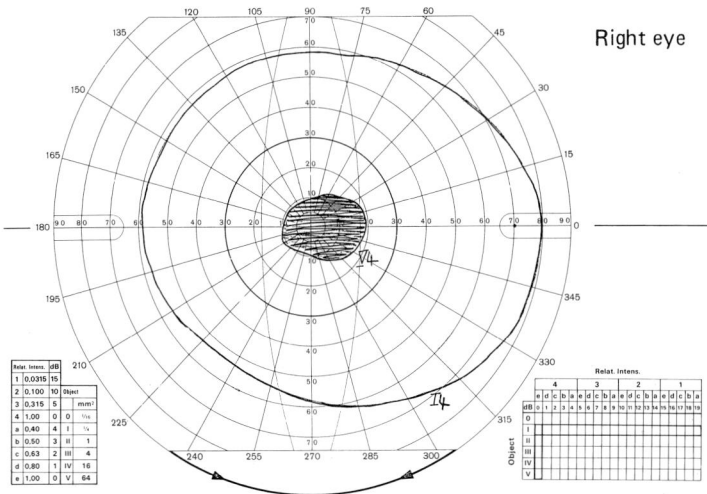

Answer to question 19

1. Right optic nerve at its junction with the chiasm.
2. Tuberculum sellae meningioma.
3. Plain skull X-ray and and CT scanning.

This patient had accidentally discovered that she had become blind in the right eye on covering her left eye. Compressive lesions of the posterior part of the optic nerve produce a central scotoma as the papillomacular bundle is most sensitive to pressure. The contralateral lower nasal fibres, which sweep forwards into the optic nerve before passing posteriorly as the anterior knee of Willibrand, may also become involved, producing a contralateral upper temporal defect (together known as a junctional field defect). For this reason all patients with unilateral visual loss should have a careful visual field examination of the opposite eye.

Abnormalities on plain skull X-ray are seen in a high proportion of cases with meningiomas and include hyperostosis, abnormal bone texture, blistering, erosion and calcification. On CT scanning they appear as contrast-enhancing masses which may be difficult to differentiate from aneurysms, in which case arteriography is indicated.

Compressive optic neuropathy may also be produced by pituitary tumours, craniopharyngiomas, aneurysms and meningiomas at other sites (optic nerve sheath, sphenoid wing).

Question 20

This fit 53-year-old woman complained of a gradual reduction of visual acuity of the right eye over about three years.

What is the most likely diagnosis?

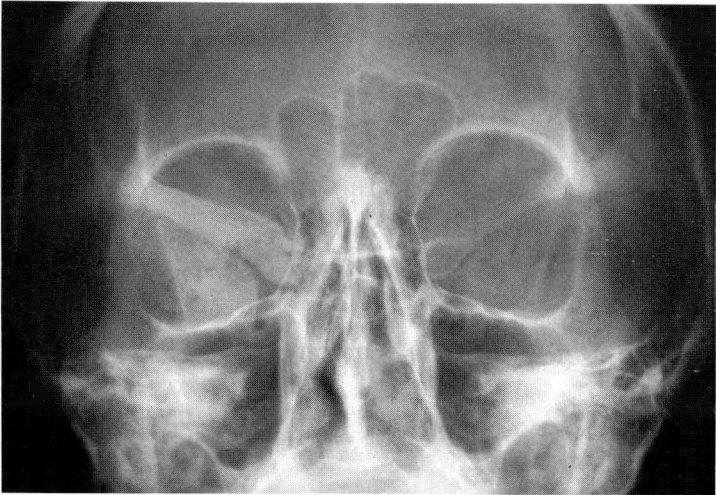

Answer to question 20

Sphenoid wing meningioma.

Meningiomas are benign tumours arising from the arachnoid mater. They account for 15% of all primary intracranial tumours. Patients usually present in their sixth decade, females being affected more often than males. Sphenoid wing meningiomas may present with symptoms of optic nerve compression, proptosis, or fullness of the temporal fossa. The diagnosis is confirmed from plain skull X-rays and CT scan which shows hyperostosis or other changes of bone texture, e.g. erosion, blistering and calcification. The differential diagnosis in this case includes sarcoma and metastatic carcinoma.

In many cases no treatment is indicated, although resection of the tumour using an operating microscope may be carried out.

Question 21

This 65-year-old man presented with intermittent diplopia.

1. What is the likely diagnosis?
2. How might you confirm the diagnosis?

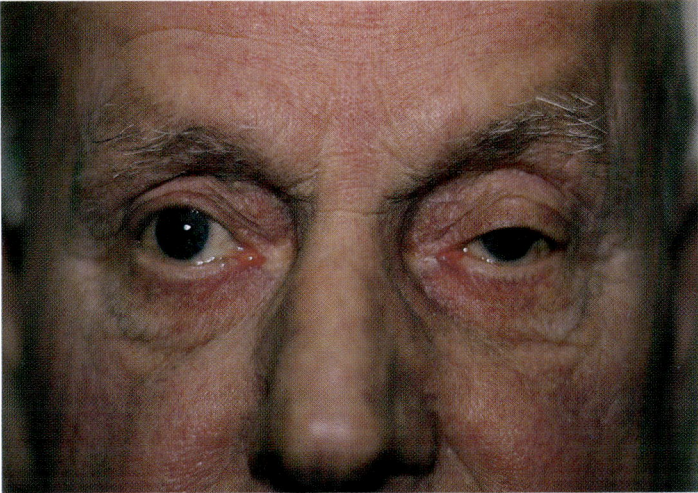

Answer to question 21

1. Myasthenia gravis.
2. (a) Tensilon test.
   (b) Detection of acetyl choline receptor antibodies.
   (c) Electromyography.

Myasthenia gravis is an immunological disorder of neuromuscular transmission in which antibodies bind to striated muscle acetylcholine receptors in such a way as to block the normal binding of acetylcholine to the muscle receptors. Although any skeletal muscle group may be affected, the disease most commonly affects the extraocular muscles and presents with ocular symptoms, usually diplopia and ptosis, in 50% of cases. If the disease is limited to the extraocular muscles it is termed ocular myasthenia. It may manifest in a wide variety of ways and can mimic a III (pupil sparing), IV or VI nerve palsy, gaze palsy, internuclear ophthalmoplegia, or other abnormalities of ocular movement. Clinically the hallmark of the disease is fatigability on sustained upgaze or lateral gaze. Patients with ocular myasthenia which does not progress to systemic involvement within two years have an 80% chance that the disease will remain localised.

The Tensilon test involves the intravenous administration of edrophonium, a short-acting anticholinesterase agent, which increases acetyl choline at the receptor site, improving muscle function. Clinically this can be observed by monitoring an improvement in ptosis or extraocular muscle movement. Acetyl choline receptor antibodies are found in 60–90% of patients with myasthenia gravis and are diagnostic of the disease. They are seen less often in ocular myasthenia but their absence does not rule out the diagnosis. The EMG has a characteristic appearance of a rapid reduction of muscle action potentials on repetitive stimulation of a peripheral nerve and may or may not be seen in ocular myasthenia.

Thyrotoxicosis develops in 5% of patients and thymic tumours (detectable on CT scanning) in 10–15%.

Acetylcholinesterase inhibitors are the mainstay of treatment often in combination with immunosuppression (corticosteroids and azathioprine). Many patients with ocular myasthenia respond poorly to conventional treatment. In patients with thymomas, thymectomy should be considered.

Question 22

1. Name three abnormalities in this fundus.
2. What is the diagnosis?

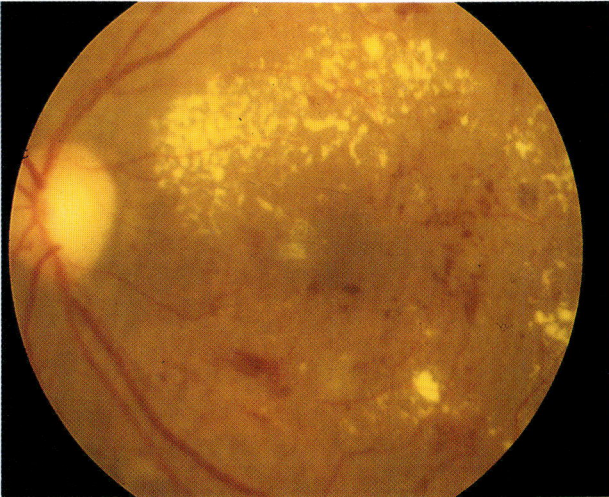

Answer to question 22

1. Microaneurysms, dot and blot haemorrhages and hard exudates.
2. Diabetic retinopathy (maculopathy).

Diabetic retinopathy is the commonest cause of blindness in the 20 to 65-year-old age group. In the majority of cases blindness is due to diabetic maculopathy with loss of central vision and preserved peripheral vision, but in others the blindness is the result of proliferative retinopathy.

Background retinopathy is the most common type of diabetic retinopathy and the visual acuity is normal in these cases. The lesions are intraretinal and most prominent in the temporal retina between the vascular arcades. Fluorescein angiography is helpful in evaluating patients with retinopathy and will show the extent of retinal ischaemia. No treatment is indicated apart from good diabetic control and treatment of any associated hypertension.

Involvement of the macula, however, leads to reduced visual acuity and is more common in maturity-onset diabetes. The poor vision may result from hard exudates or ischaemia at the macula or diffuse macular oedema. Some patients with maculopathy may respond to laser photocoagulation, particularly those with exudative maculopathy.

Question 23

1. What is the diagnosis?
2. How is the diagnosis made?

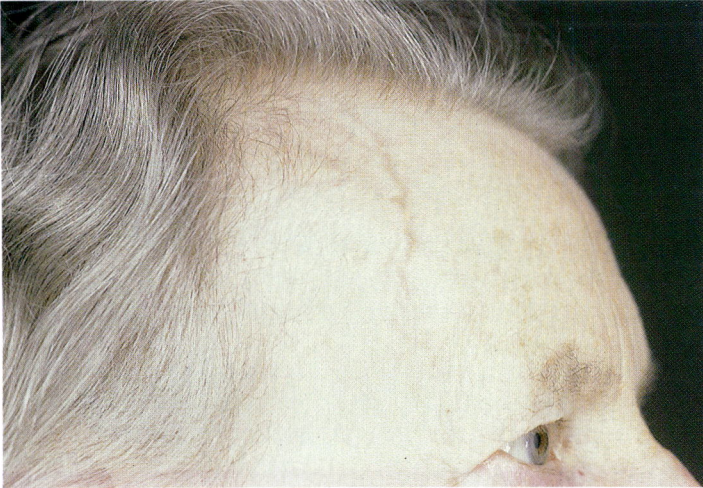

46

Answer to question 23

1. Giant cell arteritis.
2. The diagnosis is based on:
   (a) clinical signs and symptoms which include: temporal headaches, scalp tenderness, neck ache, jaw claudication, malaise, weight loss, transient loss of vision and blindness.
   (b) high erythrocyte sedimentation rate.
   (c) temporal artery biopsy — multinucleate giant cells are seen in the elastic lamina of the vessel wall.

Giant cell arteritis must always be considered in any person over 60 years of age who presents with sudden loss of vision. It is an inflammatory condition of medium-sized vessels most commonly involving the temporal arteries, but which may lead to blindness if the short posterior ciliary arteries (serving the optic disc) are affected. This occurs in about 30% of cases. Very rarely a sudden deterioration in visual acuity may be due to central retinal artery occlusion. Third and sixth cranial nerve palsies and brainstem infarction may also occur.

Polymyalgia rheumatica is commonly associated with cranial arteritis.

In the presence of appropriate clinical signs and symptoms and a high ESR treatment should be commenced immediately without awaiting the temporal artery biopsy result, as visual loss is irreversible and the other eye is at risk. Treatment should be started immediately with high-dose intravenous hydrocortisone for a duration dictated by clinical response and the ESR. Simultaneously oral prednisolone should be commenced. Steroid treatment is usually required for 1–2 years in a reducing dose which is monitored by the patient's symptoms and the ESR.

Question 24

This patient is severely incapacitated by this problem.

What is the diagnosis?

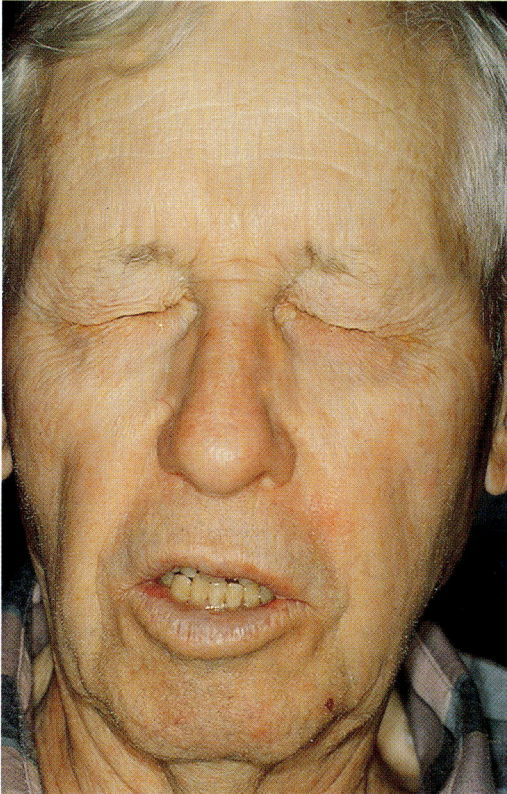

Answer to question 24

Blepharospasm.

Essential blepharospasm is a condition which most commonly presents between 45 and 60 years of age. The disorder begins with excessive blinking which progresses to total involuntary spasm of the eyelids. The disorder is usually bilateral, although it may begin unilaterally, and may be severe enough to impair vision to the extent of functional blindness. There may also be spasm of the muscles of the lower face and neck, with signs of basal ganglia dysfunction. The symptoms may be aggravated by a variety of factors including stress, speech, bright lights and fatigue. Many patients are able to initiate eye opening using physical cues such as rubbing the upper eyelid. Sometimes symptoms disappear spontaneously, but otherwise local treatment with botulinum toxin is frequently successful. The toxin is injected around the eye to paralyse the nerve fibres of the facial nerve which supply orbicularis oculi. This treatment must be repeated at regular intervals. Surgical excision of orbicularis oculi or facial nerve avulsion may be attempted in persistent cases.

Occasionally, if an underlying psychiatric disorder is present treatment with anti-depressant drugs is beneficial.

Meige's syndrome is a dystonic condition in which blepharospasm is a major feature and associated with mouth retraction, facial grimacing and jaw opening. Reflex blepharospasm is caused by ocular inflammation or referred trigeminal pain from retro-orbital or meningeal disease. Treatment is directed towards the underlying pathology.

Question 25

1. What is the diagnosis?
2. Name two ways in which this condition may affect visual acuity.

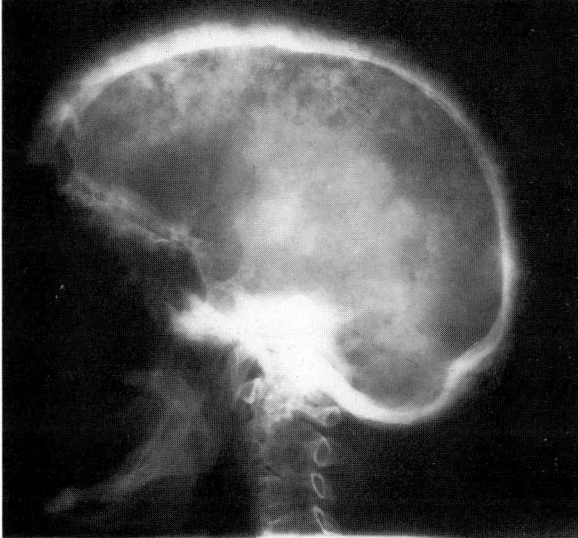

Answer to question 25

1. Paget's disease.
2. (a) Blindness due to optic nerve compression.
   (b) Angioid streaks.

Paget's disease of bone is a metabolic disorder characterised by excessive and disorganised resorption and formation of bone. The axial skeleton is commonly involved and the spinal cord is particularly at risk due to the combined effects of increased (abnormal) bone mass and vertebral collapse leading to paraplegia or corda equina lesions. Alterations of cranial bony morphology may lead to multiple cranial nerve palsies and basilar obstruction to CSF drainage and internal hydrocephalus. Although most cranial nerves can be compressed by Pagetic bone, the seventh, eighth and tenth nerves are particularly at risk. Rarely, involvement of the optic nerve may lead to optic atrophy and the association of Paget's disease with angioid streaks (linear splits in Bruch's membrane) may lead to visual loss as a result of disciform degeneration.

Question 26

These are the MRI scans of a 38-year-old man. He presented with a history of headaches and difficulty in reading which had become progressively worse over a six-month period. His pupils were unreactive to light but constricted on accommodation.

1. What abnormality is shown?
2. What syndrome is associated with this abnormality?
3. What are the three main features of this syndrome?

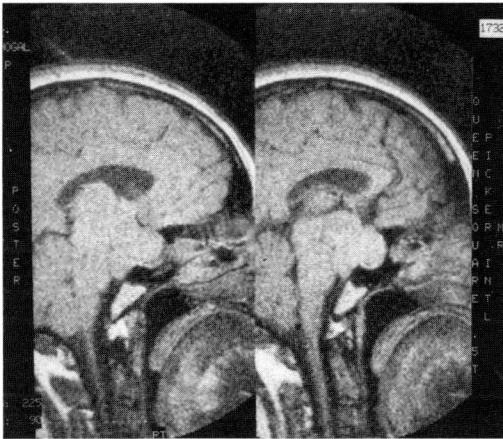

A

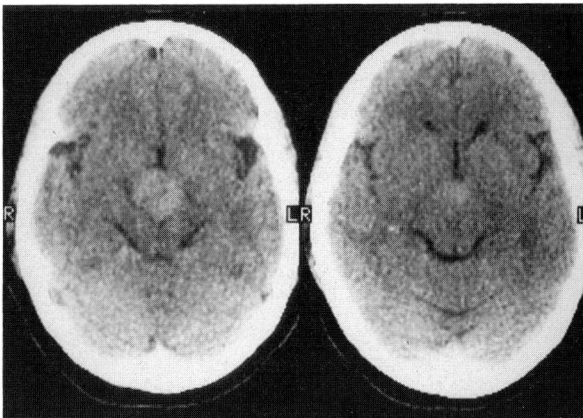

B

Answer to question 26

1. Pineal tumour.
2. Dorsal midbrain syndrome (Parinaud's syndrome).
3. (a) Convergence retraction nystagmus on attempted upgaze.
   (b) Paresis of upgaze saccades.
   (c) Pupillary light-near dissociation (dilated sluggish pupils).

Tumours, vascular lesions and demyelinating disease involving the dorsal midbrain region can all lead to this syndrome. Pinealomas are found in only a small number of cases. Initially there is loss of saccades on upgaze with retention of pursuit movement. Abnormal optokinetic nystagmus can be demonstrated when the drum is rotated downwards (due to absence of the fast phase on upgaze, i.e. saccadic phase), but when the drum is rotated up the nystagmus is normal. In progressive lesions loss of downgaze develops and eventually there follows a complete vertical gaze palsy, affecting pursuit, vestibulo-ocular movements and leading to loss of Bell's phenomenon. Convergence retraction nystagmus is best seen on testing optokinetic nystagmus, rotating the drum downwards thereby stimulating the upward refixational saccades. Upper eyelid retraction (Collier's sign) is also a feature of the syndrome and may be unilateral or bilateral.

Question 27

This woman complained of sudden severe right-sided headache and supraorbital pain.

1. What is the diagnosis?
2. What ocular signs may be detected?
3. What is the most likely cause of this lesion?

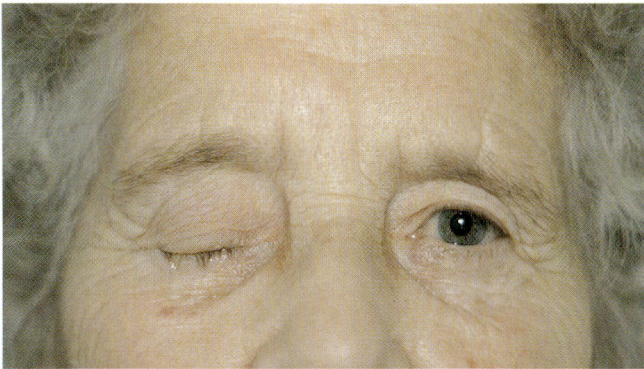

A

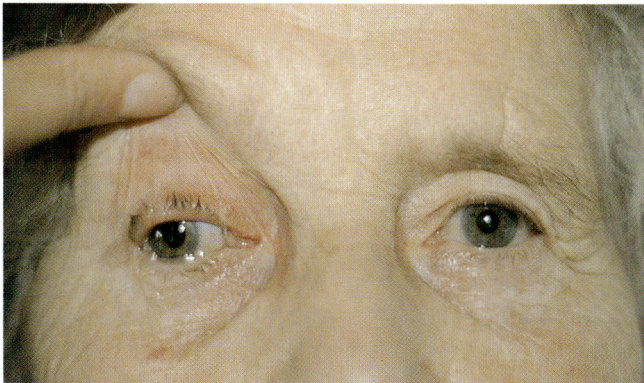

B

Answer to question 27

1. Third cranial nerve palsy.
2. (a) Ptosis — due to paralysis of levator palpebrae superioris.
   (b) Divergent squint — due to unopposed action of the superior oblique and lateral rectus muscles, rotating the eyeball laterally and downwards.
   (c) Dilatation of the pupil — the dilator action of the sympathetic fibres being unopposed.
   (d) Loss of accommodation.
3. Aneurysm of the posterior communicating artery aneurysm, near or at the bifurcation of the posterior cerebral artery.

This patient had recently bled from a posterior communicating artery aneurysm, a diagnosis suggested by the very sudden onset of symptoms, particularly the severe right-sided headache. The nucleus of the oculomotor nerve is a midline structure lying in the floor of the cerebral aqueduct at the level of the superior colliculus. It has two components: the somatic efferent nucleus supplying the extraocular muscles (except superior oblique and lateral rectus) and the Edinger–Westphal nucleus from which parasympathetic fibres pass to the sphincter pupillae via the ciliary ganglion. The efferent fibres of the oculomotor nuclei have a long intramedullary path, traversing the medial longitudinal fasiculus, red nucleus and substantia nigra before leaving the ventral surface of the brain and passing via the interpeduncular cistern, cavernous sinus and superior orbital fissure to the eye. Within the interpeduncular cistern the nerve is closely related to both the posterior cerebral and posterior communicating arteries where the peripherally situated parasympathetic pupillary fibres are readily compressed by any aneurysmal dilatation, producing a third nerve lesion with pupillary involvement. Vascular pathology such as diabetes mellitus or hypertension affecting the vasa vasorum results in infarction of the central nerve fibres along with consequent paralysis of the external ocular muscles and pupillary sparing.

Question 28

This 25-year-old man complained of visual disturbance.

What is the diagnosis?

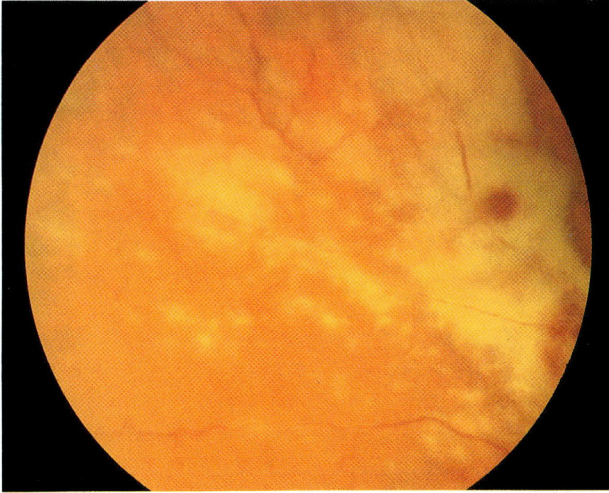

Answer to question 28

Cytomegalovirus retinal infection.

Cytomegalovirus retinitis is most commonly seen in immunocompromised individuals and is a feature of the acquired immunodeficiency syndrome (AIDS). The characteristic retinal appearance is described as 'cottage cheese and tomato sauce', due to creamy white infiltration of the retina in combination with widespread areas of retinitis and haemorrhage. Retinal involvement usually begins at the posterior pole and follows the distribution of the retinal vessels. The lesions progress slowly and vision is good unless the macula or optic nerve become involved. The development of CMV retinitis in an AIDS patient is a poor overall prognostic sign and, although the lesions may initially respond to intravenous dihydroxypropoxymethylguanine (DHPG), relapse after treatment is common.

Other ocular features of AIDS include orbital and conjunctival Kaposi's sarcoma, herpes zoster ophthalmicus, toxoplasmosis, candida and cryptococcal retinitis, multiple cotton wool spots and retinal vasculitis. Neurophthalmic manifestations include cranial nerve palsies, visual field defects and papilloedema.

Question 29

What is the diagnosis?

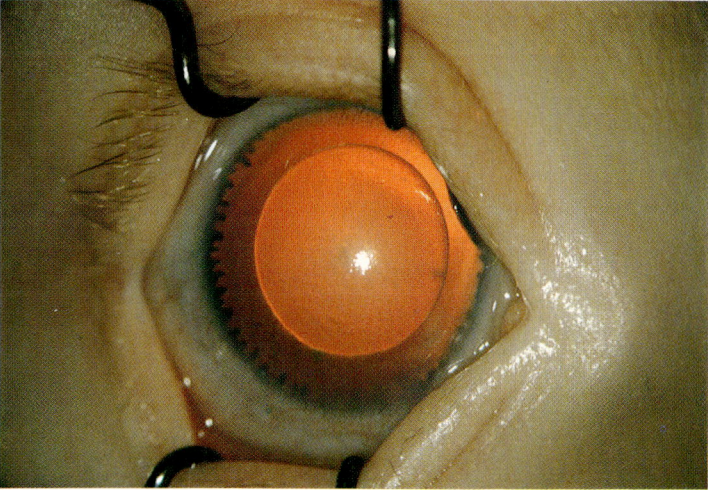

Answer to question 29

Aniridia.

Aniridia is a congenital absence of iris which is usually bilateral but may be asymmetrical. It may occur sporadically or be inherited as an autosomal dominant trait. In about 20% of sporadic cases a nephroblastoma (Wilms' tumour) may develop and this is associated with a deletion of the short arm of chromosome 11.

Glaucoma occurs in about 50% of cases and is extremely difficult to control. Other ocular features include corneal pannus, cataract, nystagmus and hypoplasia of the macula and optic nerve.

Question 30

This 50-year-old man with a longstanding ptosis but no diplopia is attempting to look up.

What is the most likely diagnosis?

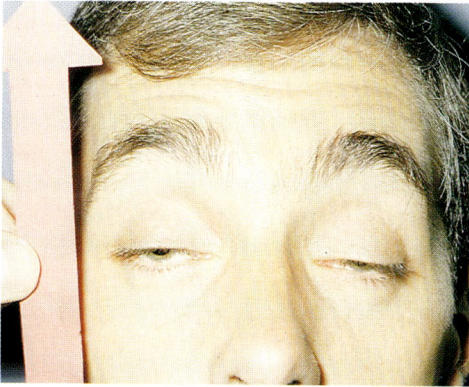

Answer to question 30

Chronic progressive external ophthalmoplegia (CPEO).

This slowly progressive myopathy affects mainly the extraocular muscles, including levator palpebrae superioris. Inheritance is autosomal dominant or recessive and onset is usually in childhood, but may be as late as 50 years of age. As the extraocular muscles are all affected simultaneously the eye remains in a central position and diplopia is not a feature. There is no muscule fatigueability and symptoms and signs remain constant throughout the day. The term CPEO is used to encompass all slowly progressive ophthalmoplegias, and may be part of a multisystem disorder. Kearns Sayre syndrome is a distinct entity with cardiac conduction defects, pigmentary retinopathy and ophthalmoplegia. The pathophysiology of many of these myopathies appears to be a defect of muscle mitochondria.

Question 31

1. List three ocular abnormalities associated with this condition.
2. How may the diagnosis be confirmed?

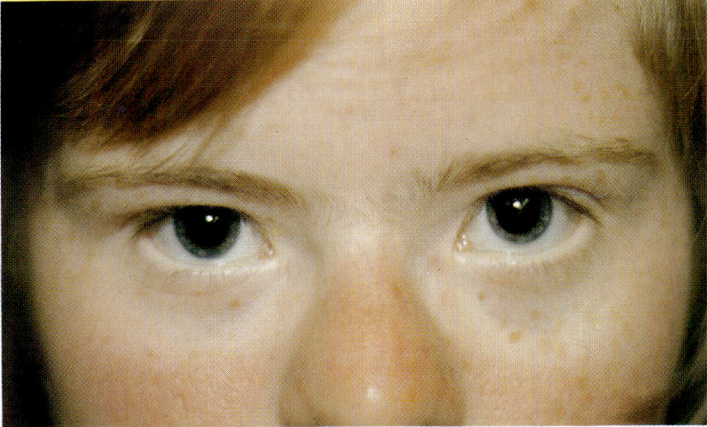

Answer to question 31

1. Ocular abnormalities include: cataracts, iris nodules (Brushfield's spots), keratoconus, blepharitis, squint and myopia.
2. Chromosomal analysis to detect trisomy 21.

Down's syndrome is recognised clinically by the characteristic features: mental deficiency, small stature, brachycephaly, epicanthic folds, short, rounded palpable apertures which slant up and outwards, and cardiac anomalies, most commonly atrial septal defects. Brushfield's spots are areas of increased density in the iris stroma seen as white or yellowish elevated spots around the periphery of the iris; they occur commonly in Down's syndrome patients and in 20% of the normal population.

Chromosomal abnormalities include anomalies of number (aneuploidy and polyploidy) and structural rearrangement of genetic material within, or between, chromosomes.

Question 32

This patient complains of pain in the left axilla and weight loss.

1. What abnormalities are shown?
2. What is the most likely underlying cause in this patient?
3. List three other causes for the abnormality shown.

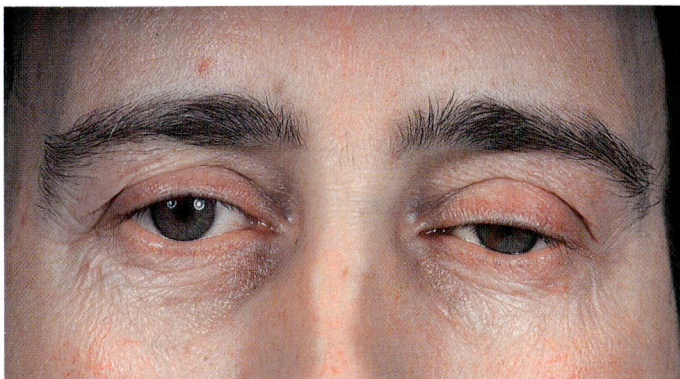

Answer to question 32

1. Enophthalmos, miosis, ptosis.
2. Pancoast's syndrome, due to an apical carcinoma of the lung.
3. (a) Unilateral massive cerebral infarction.
   (b) Brainstem lesions: infarctions, gliomas, encephalitis, multiple sclerosis.
   (c) Central cervical cord lesions: syringomyelia, gliomas, ependymomas (may cause bilateral Horner's syndrome).
   (d) Cervical damage in the neck due to thyroid or laryngeal surgery.
   (e) Malignant disease in the jugular foramen.
   (f) Congenital — usually associated with poor pigmentation of the iris.

This patient has Horner's syndrome, the features of which are ptosis, elevation of the lower eyelid, apparent enophthalmos, miosis, diminished sweating, and increased amplitude of accommodation. Horner's syndrome results from partial or total interruption of the sympathetic chain at any point from the hypothalamus to the lateral grey matter of the spinal cord at C8–T2 (first neurone) to the superior cervical ganglion (second neurone) to the pupil and blood vessels of the eye (third neurone). The diagnosis is confirmed using 4% cocaine eye drops which fail to dilate the pupil in Horner's syndrome. Preganglionic lesions may be distinguished from post-ganglionic using hydroxyamphetamine eye drops which dilate the pupil only if post-ganglionic fibres are intact. Lesions above the superior cervical ganglion do not cause anhydrosis. The patient illustrated had an apical carcinoma of the left lung which affected the second neurone of the sympathetic chain where it crosses the apical pleura.

Question 33

This 58-year-old publican presented with progressive ataxia, confusion and diplopia. He is attempting to look to the left.

1. What is the diagnosis?
2. What is the immediate management?

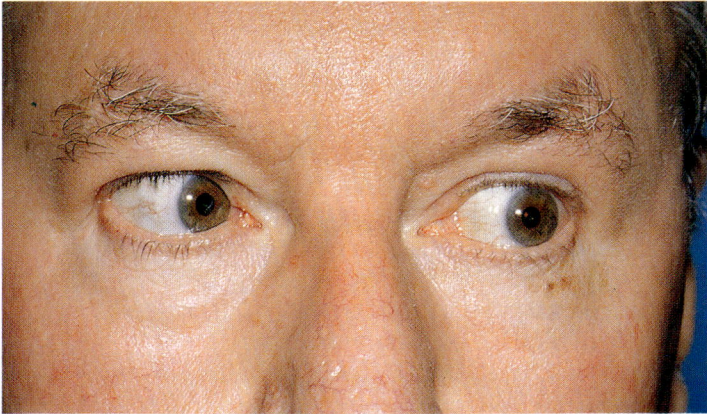

Answer to question 33

1. Wernicke's encephalopathy.
2. Intravenous thiamine.

Wernicke's encephalopathy is a neurological triad of ophthalmoplegia, ataxia and a global confusional state resulting from thiamine deficiency. In this country it is most commonly associated with chronic alcoholic abuse, but may be seen in other conditions associated with poor nutrition such as advanced carcinoma, hyperemesis gravidarum, prolonged intravenous feeding and starvation.

Ocular signs are the hallmark of Wernicke's encephalopathy and include horizontal nystagmus, bilateral VI nerve paresis, conjugate gaze palsies and less commonly pupillary abnormalities, ptosis, retinal haemorrhages and papilloedema. The confusional state is manifest by apathy, impaired memory, inability to concentrate and restlessness. Other features include coma, hypotension and hypothermia.

The neuropathological changes of the condition are characteristic with bilateral symmetrical neuronal necrosis of the mamillary bodies, superior cerebellar vermis and hypothalamic nuclei.

Early recognition of the disorder is critical as the mortality rate is 10–20% and treatment may correct all the abnormalities. Because of the high risk of sudden death the condition should be treated as a medical emergency and high-dose intravenous thiamine administered. Eighty per cent of patients who survive will have Korsakoff's psychosis, and of these 25% do not recover.

Question 34

This fit 43-year-old man with normal visual acuity presented to the out-patient clinic.

1. What abnormality is shown?
2. What ocular symptoms may have occurred?
3. List three important investigations.

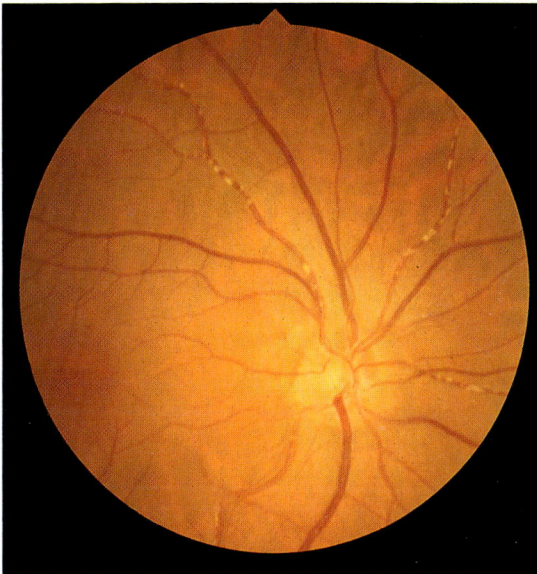

Answer to question 34

1. Cholesterol emboli (Hollenhorst plaques).
2. Transient uniocular visual loss either:
   (a) concentric peripheral dimming of vision or
   (b) a horizontal curtain coming over the eye (amaurosis fugax).
3. (a) Plasma lipid levels.
   (b) Blood pressure measurement.
   (c) Carotid artery digital subtraction angiogram.

Cholesterol crystals are a sign of atheromatous disease, usually in the carotid arteries, and are seen in elderly patients often as an incidental finding. Patients are therefore at considerable risk of developing permanent visual loss or cerebral infarction. The crystals are often multiple and are found most commonly at the bifurcations of the retinal arterioles. Most patients with cholesterol emboli are asymptomatic as retinal blood flow is usually undisturbed due to the plain shape of the crystal. In younger patients cholesterol emboli are associated with underlying disorders of liver metabolism which should be investigated.

Question 35

This 17-year-old boy presented with short stature and delayed puberty.

1. What is the diagnosis?
2. What visual field defect might be present?
3. What is the management?

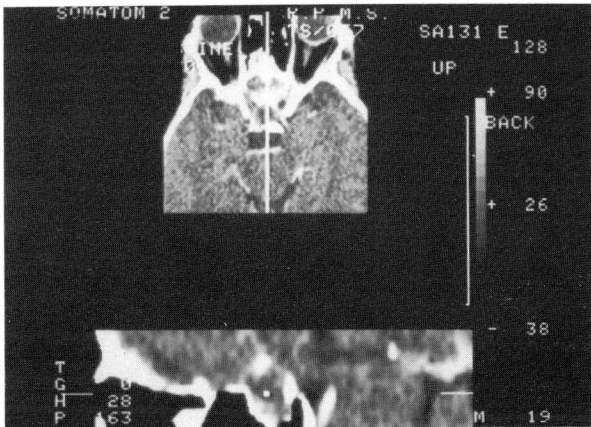

A

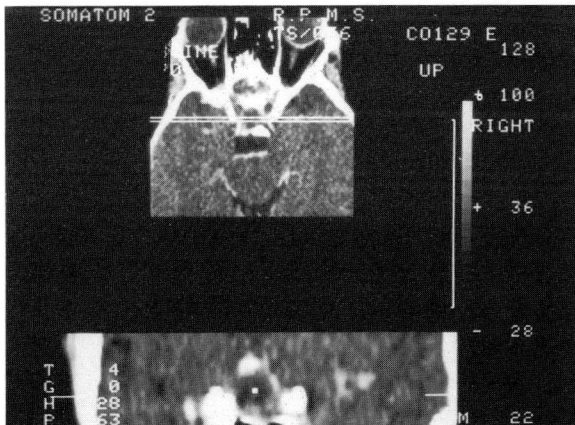

B

Answer to question 35

1. Hypopituitarism secondary to a craniopharyngioma.
2. Bitemporal hemianopia or homonymous hemianopia.
3. (a) Surgical removal followed by radiotherapy.
   (b) Hormone replacement therapy according to the post-operative dynamic pituitary function tests.

Craniopharyngiomas arise from developmental cell rests in Rathke's pouch and present as space-occupying lesions. The tumours usually develop adjacent to the optic nerve and chiasm and may invade the third ventricle or extend into the cerebral hemispheres. They most commonly present in childhood or adolescence with obesity, failure of growth, delayed sexual development and diabetes insipidus, or hydrocephalus due to obstruction of the third ventricle. In older patients raised intracranial pressure and mental deterioration may occur. The visual pathways may become involved, leading to visual failure (optic nerve involvement), homonymous hemianopia (optic tract involvement) or bitemporal field defect (optic chiasm involvement). In adults, 50% of tumours are large calcified cystic masses, but do not usually invade the pituitary fossa.

Question 36

1. What is the diagnosis?
2. What abnormality might you see on fundal examination?

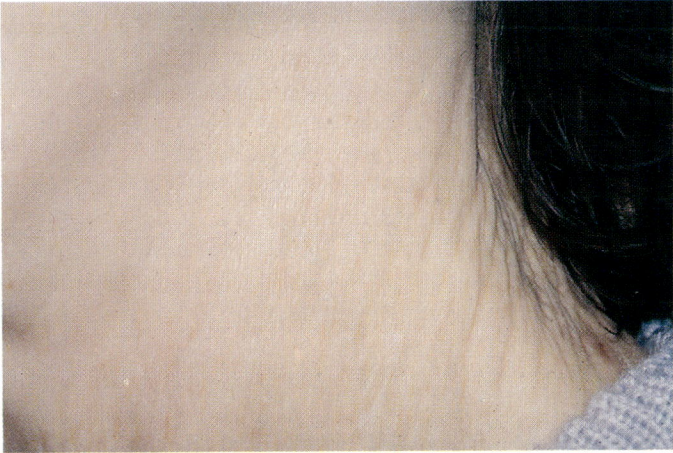

Answer to question 36

1. Pseudoxanthoma elasticum.
2. Angioid streaks.

Pseudoxanthoma elasticum is an inherited disorder of elastic tissue of which there are four distinct types:

(a) Dominant type 1: skin involvement, severe degeneration of Bruch's membrane leading to early blindness, vascular complications and coronary artery disease.

(b) Dominant type 2: mild vascular and retinal involvement, but blue sclerae and myopia occur.

(c) Recessive type 1: similar to (a), but mild retinal involvement.

(d) Recessive type 2: skin involvement only.

Question 37

This patient complained of diplopia and numbness of his left cheek which were persistent after an assault 10 days before.

1. What is the diagnosis?
2. Why does he complain of numbness of his cheek?

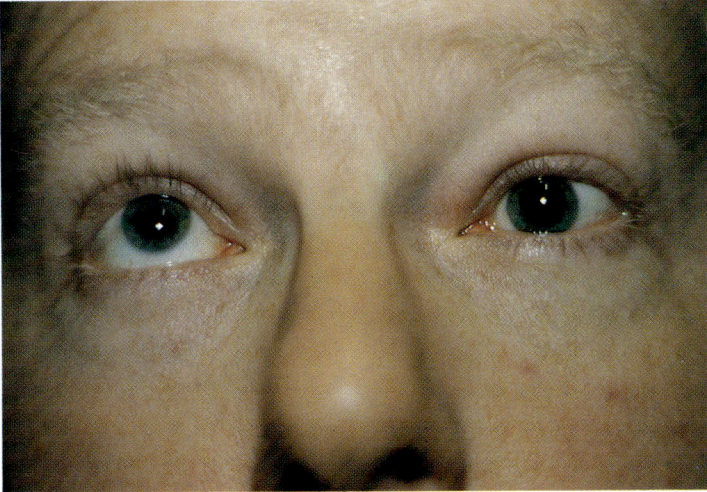

Answer to question 37

1. Orbital blow-out fracture.
2. Contusion of the infraorbital nerve.

Blunt trauma to the orbit by an object such as a fist or a ball
may result in a fracture of the orbital wall and not the orbital
rim. The orbital floor (maxillary bone) and the medial wall
(ethmoid bone) are most frequently involved. Limitation of
upgaze and downgaze may be due to entrapment of orbital
tissues or extraocular muscles, oedema or haemorrhage in the
surrounding tissues. The infraorbital nerve which passes
through a canal in the orbital floor may be contused causing
numbness of the cheek and incisor area of the upper jaw. Other
signs of a blow-out fracture include enophthalmos due to
herniation of orbital contents into the maxillary sinus, bruising
of the lids, subconjunctival haemorrhage and surgical
emphysema, especially after blowing the nose. All patients with
orbital fractures must have a thorough ocular examination to
exclude associated ocular trauma. This patient has a traumatic
mydriasis of his left pupil which should be differentiated from a
III nerve palsy.

The diagnosis can be confirmed radiologically with tilted P-A
skull X-rays which may show the fracture, herniation of tissue
or a fluid level in the maxillary sinus. Orbital tomography and
computerised tomography are useful in suspicious cases.

Most patients recover spontaneously within the first
2–3 weeks but surgery may be indicated in those with
troublesome diplopia or enophthalmos.

Question 38

What is the diagnosis?

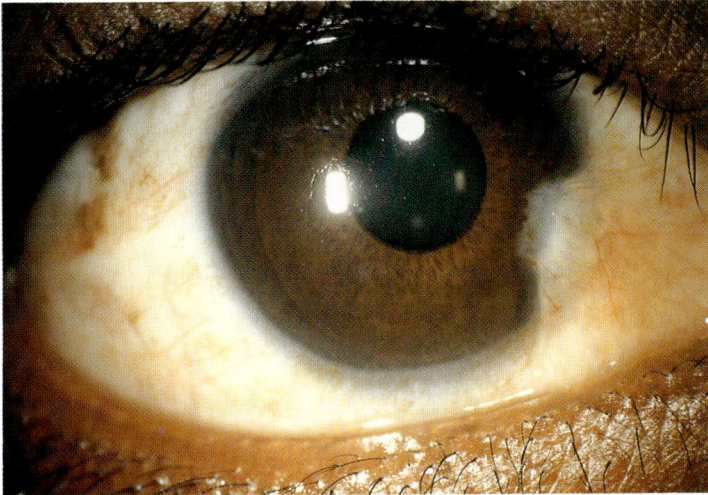

Answer to question 38

Pterygium.

Pterygia begin as a degenerative change of the conjunctiva which encroach onto the cornea in a triangular fashion occurring initially on the nasal side and later on the temporal side of the cornea. They are seen most commonly in individuals living in hot climates and are thought to be associated with chronic exposure to the sun. Many patients complain of mild irritation but surgical excision is indicated only in those cases where the pterygium has encroached onto the visual axis and affected vision, but the recurrence rate after surgery is high.

Question 39

This 20-year-old woman described an eight-month history of headaches and a four-week history of blackouts of vision lasting for a few seconds. Neurological examination and a CT scan were normal.

What is the diagnosis?

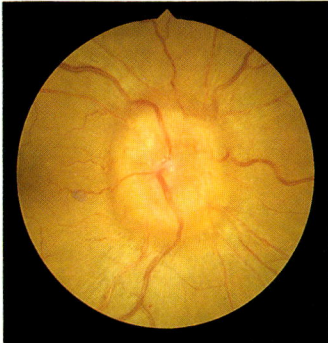 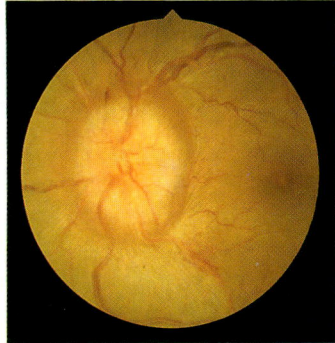

RIGHT EYE   LEFT EYE

Answer to question 39

Benign intracranial hypertension (pseudotumour cerebri).

Bilateral papilloedema in the presence of a normal CT scan and in the absence of focal neurological signs is nearly always due to benign intracranial hypertension (BIH), although it may be mimicked by dural venous sinus thrombosis. The disorder is most common in otherwise healthy obese young women but has been associated with drug therapy (tetracyclines, nalidixic acid, steroid withdrawal), vitamin A intoxication, systemic lupus erythematosis and renal failure.

Symptoms include headache, transient visual obscurations, blurred vision, diplopia and less commonly tinnitus, facial pain and neck pain. Although termed benign, serious visual loss occurs in 25% of patients. In the early stages there is enlargement of the blind spot, but visual field defects develop usually in a nerve fibre bundle distribution, and extensive field loss may occur before visual acuity is affected. Diplopia, when present, is due to involvement of the VI nerve which is a non-localising sign of raised intracranial pressure.

Treatment is indicated in those patients with transient obscurations of vision and loss of visual field as documented by perimetry. All patients should be encouraged to lose weight and be commenced on acetazolamide (Diamox®), or frusemide in patients intolerant to this. In patients with progressive visual loss despite medical therapy surgery should be considered. Optic nerve sheath decompression, in which a window is cut in the sheath of the optic nerve, is now the procedure of choice and the papilloedema resolves even though the intracranial pressure remains elevated. Lumbar–peritoneal shunting is an alternative surgical approach.

Question 40

This is the CT scan of a 40-year-old woman who presented with a five-week history of blurring of vision and loss of colour vision.

1. What is the diagnosis?
2. What is the reason for her reduced vision?

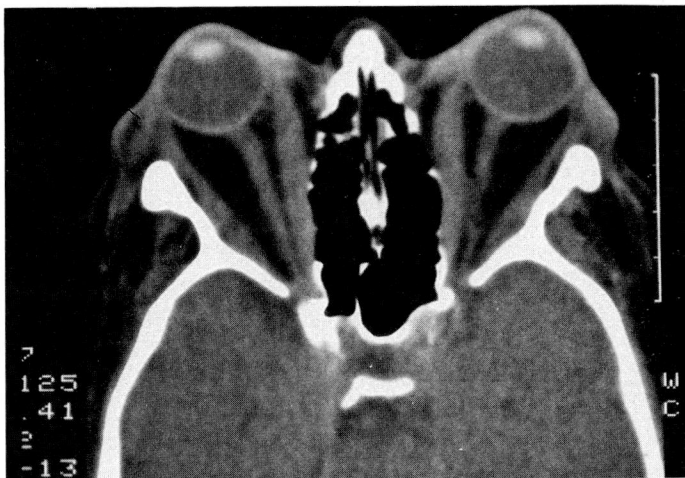

Answer to question 40

1. Dysthyroid eye disease (Graves' ophthalmopathy).
2. Compressive optic neuropathy.

Patients with thyroid eye disease may lose vision from compression of the optic nerve at the apex of the orbit by the enlarged muscles. It is more likely to occur in patients without proptosis, as those with proptosis tend to decompress their own orbits. Physical signs suggestive of optic nerve compression include decreased visual acuity, impaired colour vision, an afferent pupillary defect, visual field defects and optic disc swelling or atrophy (though the disc may be normal). CT scanning will show the enlarged muscles, most commonly medial and inferior rectus.

If patients are treated promptly visual recovery is possible. Many patients respond to high-dose systemic steroids combined with control of any thyroid dysfunction. In those cases which fail to respond to medical treatment surgical decompression of the orbit is indicated. Orbital radiation is an alternative therapy, particularly in patients at high risk from surgery.

Other causes of reduced vision in thyroid eye disease include corneal exposure, which may lead to corneal ulceration, particularly in acute disease, and secondary hypermetropia resulting from compression of the globe by the raised intraorbital pressure.

Question 41

1. What is the diagnosis?
2. Name two causes.

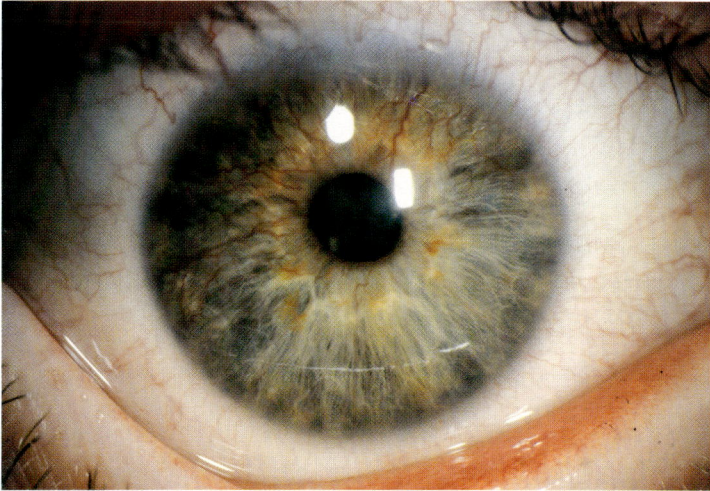

Answer to question 41

1. Rubeosis iridis.
2. (a) Proliferative diabetic retinopathy.
   (b) Central retinal vein occlusion.
   (c) Other causes: carotid ischaemia, longstanding retinal detachment, intraocular tumours, diffuse retinal vascular disease, e.g sickle cell retinopathy and retinopathy of prematurity.

Proliferative diabetic retinopathy and central retinal vein occlusion are by far the commonest causes of rubeosis iridis; all other causes are rare. In the early stages fine new vessels are seen in the anterior chamber angle and around the pupil; as the neovascularisation progresses the anterior chamber angle becomes occluded by fibrovascular tissue resulting in glaucoma and corneal oedema. It is probable that retinal hypoxia is the trigger to new vessel formation, possibly by release of an angiogenic substance.

Panretinal photocoagulation and retinal cryotherapy may cause regression of the new vessels early in the condition. Treatment in established cases is difficult, as they respond poorly to surgical treatment such as trabeculectomy and other drainage procedures. In those cases with no vision in which pain is a prominent feature topical steroids and atropine usually control the symptoms even though the pressure may remain high. In intractable cases enucleation of the eye may be necessary for pain relief.

Question 42

This child was noted at preschool screening to have reduced vision in the right eye.

1. What abnormality is shown?
2. Name two possible causes for the reduced vision.

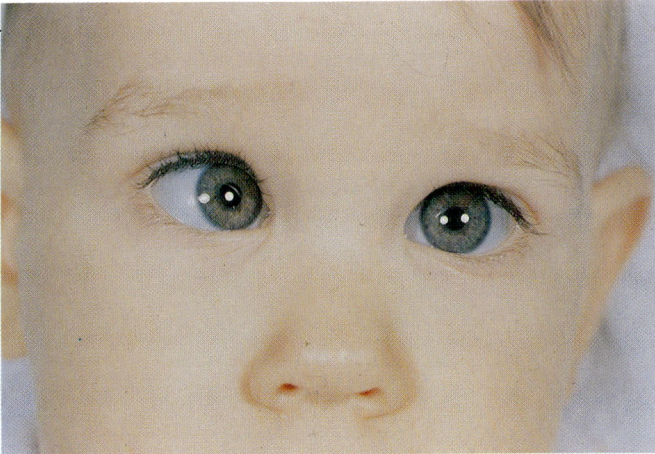

Answer to question 42

1. A right convergent squint.
2. Strabismic amblyopia, anisometropia and monocular ocular pathology.

Convergent squints in children may present in the first six months of life (infantile esotropia); the squint is typically large and requires surgical correction. In older children uncorrected hypermetropia may lead to an accommodative esotropia which may be corrected by spectacles. If there is a large difference in the refractive error of the eyes anisometropic amblyopia may result. Children with monocular organic lesions such as cataract, optic atrophy or retinoblastoma may also develop convergent squints. All children with squints must have mydriatic fundoscopy performed and their refractive error assessed.

Question 43

1. What is this investigation?
2. What abnormalities are shown?

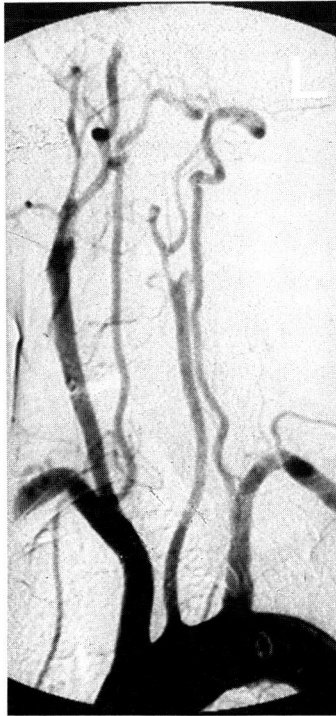

Answer to question 43

1. Digital subtraction angiography (DSA).
2. (a) Narrowing of the entire length of the left common carotid artery.
   (b) Stenosis of the origin of the left external carotid artery.
   (c) Occlusion of the left internal carotid artery just distal to its origin.
   (d) Narrowing and irregularity of the right internal and external carotid arteries.

DSA is an angiographic technique in which unwanted background bone images can be eliminated from images. Digital i.v. angiography requires large volumes of contrast media. Intra-arterial angiography provides high-contrast images with small amounts of dye, and for this reason is generally thought to be safer than conventional angiographic techniques.

Question 44

1. What does the slide show?
2. List three causes for this lesion.

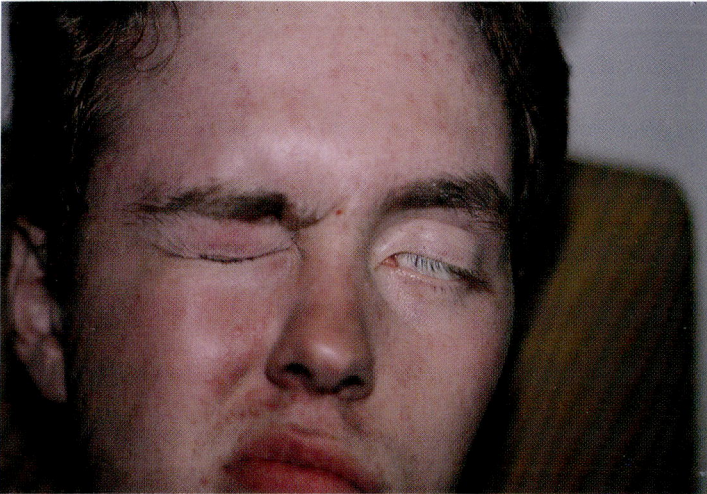

Answer to question 44

1. Lower motor neurone lesion of the left seventh cranial nerve. Bell's phenomenon (upgaze of left eye on attempted eye closure) is demonstrated.

2. Causes include: idiopathic Bell's palsy, diabetes, hypertension, middle ear disease, cholesteatoma, herpes zoster infection, Guillain–Barré syndrome, basal skull fracture, sarcoidosis, carotid tumour, brainstem lesion, pregnancy, cerebello-pontine angle tumour, multiple sclerosis and Melkersson's syndrome.

Bell's palsy describes unilateral facial paralysis of rapid onset, frequently heralded by transient facial pain below the ear. Paralysis is maximal at 2–3 days before slowly improving, with full recovery occurring within a few weeks in the majority of cases. In severe cases taste subserved by the anterior two-thirds of the tongue may be affected and paralysis of the stapedius muscle may cause hyperacusis. Paralysis of the orbicularis oculi leads to weakness of eyelid closure and an exposure keratitis may result. In patients with a good Bell's phenomenon (elevation of the eye on eyelid closure) the risk of corneal exposure is greatly diminished. Guillain–Barré syndrome and sarcoidosis are the commonest causes of bilateral seventh nerve palsies. Corneal exposure may lead to serious complications including corneal ulceration and perforation. All cases should be treated with topical ocular lubricants and if recovery is poor in the presence of significant corneal exposure then tarsorraphy should be performed.

Question 45

1. What abnormality is shown?
2. Name two systemic diseases associated with this abnormality.

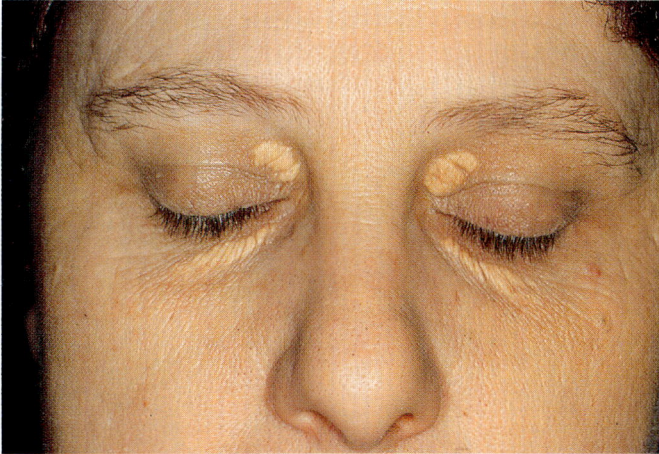

Answer to question 45

1. Eyelid xanthelasma.
2. Hyperlipidaemia, myxoedema, diabetes mellitus, primary biliary cirrhosis.

Eyelid xanthelasmata are are skin deposits of cholesterol and classically occur on the inner aspect of the upper and lower lids. Approximately 50% of patients have hyperlipidaemia with raised serum cholesterol (hyperlipidaemia types II and IV) and myxoedema, diabetes mellitus and primary biliary cirrhosis are associated. Serum lipids should therefore be be measured, especially in young patients who may have an underlying metabolic disorder. Cosmetic surgical excision of the xanthelasmata may be performed.

Question 46

This is the optic disc of a 30-year-old man with a five-day history of blurring of vision of the left eye associated with pain on ocular movement. His visual acuity was reduced in the left eye, colour vision was impaired and he had a left afferent pupillary defect.

1. What visual field defect would you expect to see?
2. What is the diagnosis?

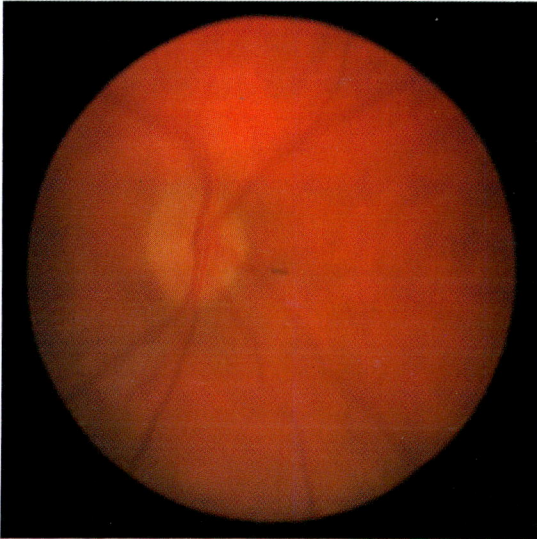

Answer to question 46

1. A left central scotoma.
2. Optic neuritis.

Optic neuritis is caused by local inflammation of the optic nerve head and is associated with optic nerve damage (reduced visual acuity, impaired colour vision, an afferent pupillary defect and a central scotoma). It is usually associated with retrobulbar pain which is exacerbated by ocular movement, which may precede or coincide with the visual loss. The appearance of the optic disc is indistinguishable from early papilloedema but the latter is not associated with optic nerve dysfunction, unless longstanding, and on visual field testing a large blind spot may be seen. In some cases of optic neuritis the optic disc appears normal as the inflammation involves the optic nerve posterior to the disc (retrobulbar neuritis). Vision may be severely affected but in most cases vision begins to improve one to several weeks after the onset, although some signs of optic nerve dysfunction persist and pallor of the disc often develops.

Acute optic neuritis is most commonly due to multiple sclerosis and may follow a viral illness. Conditions which should be considered in the differential diagnosis include sphenoid sinus mucocele, vasculitis and infiltration of the nerve with a granulomatous, carcinomatous or lymphoreticular process.

Question 47

This is the corneal appearance of a 29-year-old man receiving treatment for a cardiac arrhythmia.

1. What is the diagnosis?
2. What is the likely cause in this case?

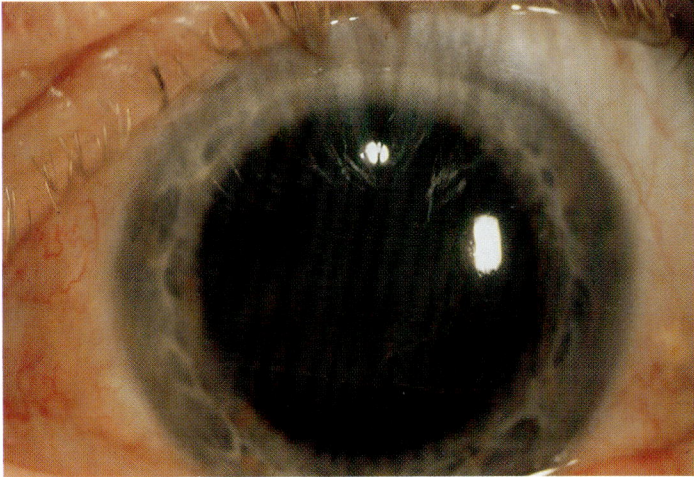

Answer to question 47

1. Corneal verticillata.
2. Amioderone therapy.

Corneal verticillata describes whorl-like corneal opacities in the subepithelial layers. There are a number of drugs that can produce this picture which include amioderone, chloroquine, indomethacin and chlorpromazine. It can also be seen in Fabry's disease, a lysosomal storage disorder. The corneal lesions do not affect vision and usually resolve when the drug is stopped.

Question 48

This 36-year-old woman presented with a slowly progressive proptosis of the left eye with no other ocular abnormalities.

What one investigation would you perform?

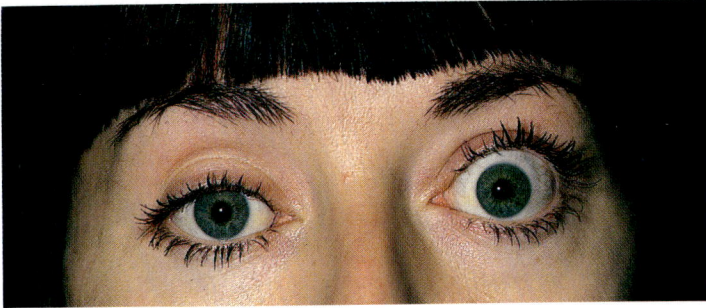

Answer to question 48

CT scan of the orbits.

CT scanning is now the investigation of choice in the management of patients with orbital disease. With the use of conventional as well as axial and coronal images the diagnosis can be established in the majority of patients with proptosis.

The commonest cause of unilateral proptosis in an adult is thyroid eye disease, and in such cases there may be other physical signs which will provide a clue to the diagnosis. Other causes of unilateral proptosis include orbital tumours, most commonly cavernous haemangioma, lymphoma, lacrimal gland tumours and in children rhabdomyosarcoma. Secondary involvement of orbital tissue by malignant disease may result from systemic metastases or local invasion by nasopharyngeal carcinomas. Orbital vascular lesions leading to proptosis include caroticocavernous fistulae and orbital varices. Inflammatory lesions may also cause proptosis and include orbital pseudotumour and conditions such as Wegener's granulomatosis. Dermoid cysts are usually seen in young adults and children but may present at any age.

Question 49

1. What is the diagnosis?
2. What precautions can be taken to avoid this situation?

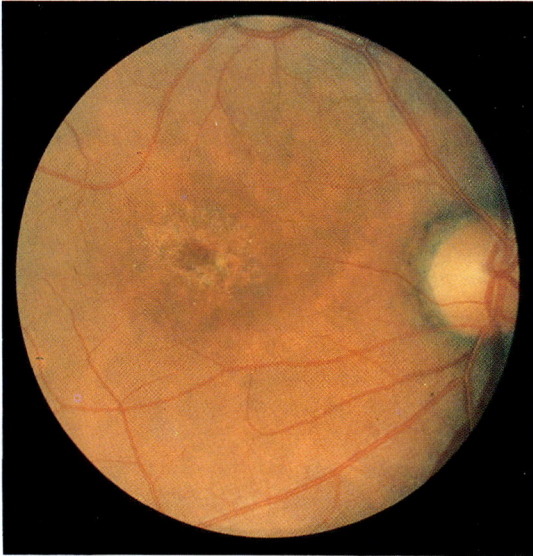

Answer to question 49

1. Chloroquine-induced 'bull's-eye' maculopathy.
2. (a) Regular ocular examination to detect the pre-maculopathy stage.
   (b) Reduce or stop chloroquine when maculopathy toxicity is first noticed.
   (c) Hydroxychloroquine is a safer drug and should be used in place of chloroquine.

Chloroquine is an anti-malarial drug, but may also be used in the long-term treatment of rheumatoid arthritis and systemic lupus erythematosis. It is excreted slowly and becomes concentrated in the melanin-containing structures of the eye, which are the choroid and retinal pigment epithelium. The incidence of retinotoxicity is dose-dependent and is rare if the total dose used does not exceed 300 g.

Ophthalmoscopy, fundal photography, and examination of colour vision, visual acuity and visual fields to a red target are essential prior to starting therapy. Examination must be repeated regularly to detect the pre-maculopathy stage, when a scotoma to a red target may be found at between four and nine degrees of fixation. Complete resolution is possible at this stage following cessation of therapy. If treatment is continued a maculopathy develops, characterised by blurring of vision, central scotoma to white objects, loss of the foveal reflex and non-specific pigment stippling of the retina. Improvement is rare despite chloroquine withdrawal at this stage and the patient may be left with irreversible impairment of peripheral and central vision which may progress. There is no correlation between the corneal deposition of chloroquine and the retinotoxic effects of this drug.

Question 50

This obese young man complained of progressive visual disturbance.

1. What is the most likely diagnosis?
2. What is the cause of his visual disturbance?
3. List two other associated features of this condition.

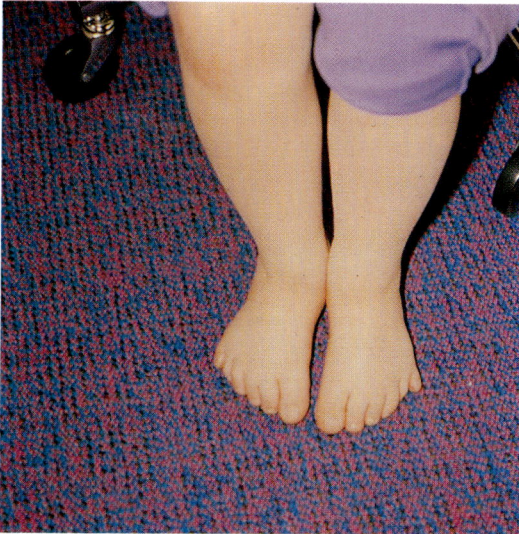

Answer to question 50

1. Laurence–Moon–Biedl syndrome.
2. Retinitis pigmentosa.
3. Hypogonadism, mental retardation, truncal obesity.

Please see question 84 for discussion of retinitis pigmentosa.

Question 51

This slit-lamp photograph shows increased iris transillumination.

1. What is the diagnosis?
2. Name two ocular abnormalities associated with this condition.

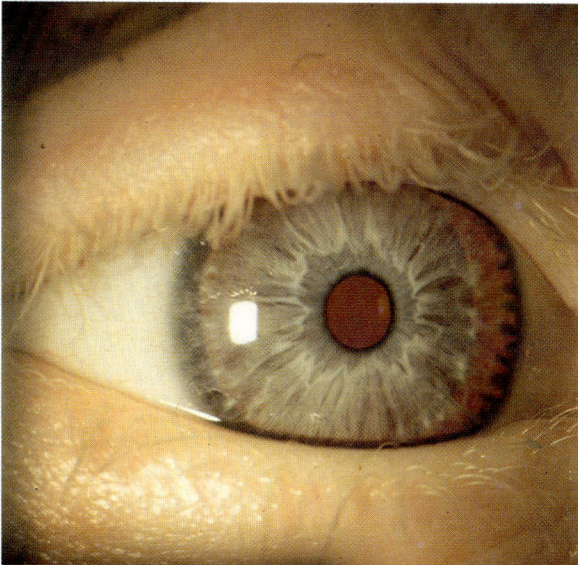

Answer to question 51

1. Albinism.
2. (a) Increased iris transillumination.
   (b) Congenital nystagmus.
   (c) Squint and amblyopia.
   (d) Hypopigmented fundi and hypoplasia of the macula.
   (e) Photophobia.
   (f) Visual acuity of 6/60 or less.
   (g) Abnormal distribution of fibres in the optic chiasm with 90% of optic nerve fibres decussating.

Albinism is an inherited defect of melanin production. There are two main types, oculocutaneous albinism and ocular albinism; the ocular features of both are indistinguishable.

Oculocutaneous albinism is most commonly an autosomal recessive condition and affects the skin, hair and eyes. There are two main subgroups of patients; tyrosinase-positive, who can synthesise variable amounts of melanin and have some pigmentation, and tyrosinase-negative, who produce no melanin. Clinically carrier detection is not usually possible in this form of albinism.

In ocular albinism the melanin deficiency is predominantly uveal and affected individuals have normal skin and hair. It is an X-linked disorder and asymptomatic female carriers may show iris transillumination and pigmentary changes in the peripheral retina.

Diagnosis of the exact type of albinism is important in order to provide accurate genetic counselling for affected families.

Question 52

This painless swelling developed in a nine-month-old boy.

1. What is the diagnosis?
2. What is the management?

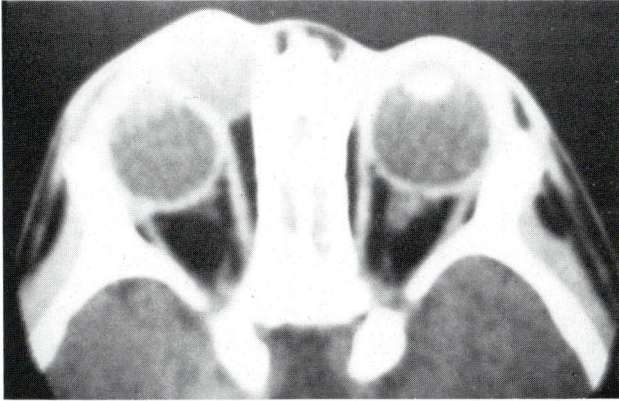

A

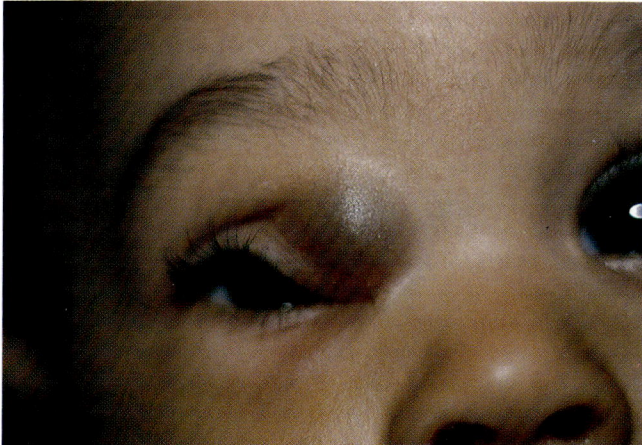

B

Answer to question 52

1. Dermoid cyst.
2. Surgical excision.

Dermoid cysts are one of the commonest tumours of childhood although they may not present until early adult life. They usually arise adjacent to bony suture lines and are thought to be formed by inclusion of surface ectoderm into the mesenchyme along embryonic facial clefts. Most dermoids are superficial and lie in the superior orbit, anterior to the orbital septum. Less commonly they lie deep to the septum and may present with proptosis; rarely they may extend intracranially and careful preoperative assessment is therefore essential.

They usually present as an asymptomatic mass in childhood but vision may be impaired by amblyopia (visual deprivation or astigmatic), optic nerve compression or choroidal folds.

Radiological assessment is essential in all cases. Plain skull X-ray may show localised bone erosion with a clearly defined sclerotic margin; CT scanning and MRI scanning will show the extent of the tumour. Orbital dermoids should be excised because they progressively enlarge, and rupture of the cyst provokes a severe inflammatory reaction. The cysts should be removed in their entirety as remnants produce a chronic inflammatory reaction.

Question 53

1. What is the diagnosis?
2. What test may aid your clinical diagnosis?

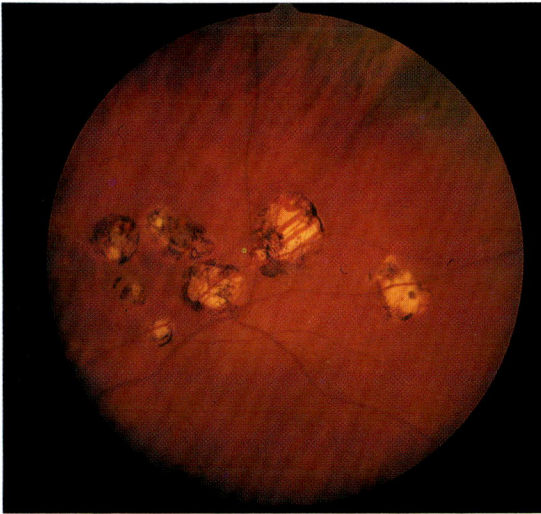

Answer to question 53

1. Toxoplasmosis retinochoroiditis.
2. A serological test for *Toxoplasma gondii.*

Toxoplasma gondii is an obligate intracellular parasite, which reproduces in the cat intestine and is shed in cat faeces. Ocular toxoplasmosis is nearly always congenital in origin; the organism crosses the placenta if a non-immune mother acquires the infection during pregnancy. Acute infection during the first trimester may result in fetal death or CNS damage, leading to convulsions, mental retardation, hydrocephalus, microcephaly and intracranial calcification which may be seen on skull X-ray. Most commonly maternal infections are subclinical and the only manifestations of infection are the healed chorioretinal scars. The parasite has a predilection for the nerve fibre layer of the retina and cysts containing the protozoa remain dormant and inactive. Recurrence usually takes place between the ages of 10 and 35 years, when the cysts rupture and release the protozoa. The protozoa then incite a severe inflammatory reaction in the retina, which is seen clinically as a focal area of necrotising retinitis adjacent to an area of previous chorioretinal scarring. These lesions heal over several months leaving atrophic scars with pigmented borders. Visual acuity may be reduced if a lesion threatens the macula, papillomacular bundle or the optic nerve head, or if there is an associated severe vitritis. In such cases treatment is indicated. The antimicrobial drugs used include clindamycin, sulphonamides and pyrimethamine, and systemic corticosteroids are added to suppress the inflammatory reaction.

Acquired toxoplasmosis is usually subclinical but may produce a glandular fever-like illness.

Question 54

1. What clinical signs are shown?
2. What is the diagnosis?
3. List two ocular and two neurological manifestations associated with this condition.

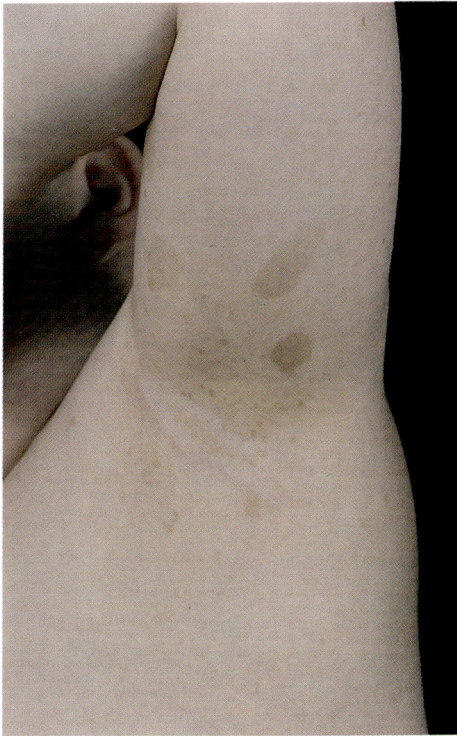

Answer to question 54

1. Café au lait spots and axillary freckles.
2. Neurofibromatosis (Von Recklinghausen's disease).
3. (a) Ocular: Lisch nodules (neurofibroma of the iris), plexiform neuroma of the eyelid, congenital glaucoma. Proptosis may occur secondary to an optic nerve glioma, orbital tumour (neurilemmoma, plexiform neuroma, meningioma) or a spheno-orbital encephalocele.
   (b) Neurological: optic nerve glioma, Schwannoma and meningioma, acoustic neuroma, spinal meningioma, mental retardation and epilepsy.

Neurofibromatosis is a phakomatosis with an incidence of 1:2500–3000 live births. It is usually of autosomal dominant inheritance with incomplete penetrance and variable expressivity, but can arise as a spontaneous mutation. The commonest clinical abnormalities are café au lait spots (areas of cutaneous hyperpigmentation) and multiple subcutaneous neurofibromata. Axillary freckles are pathognomonic.

Neurofibromatous lesions are also seen in the gastrointestinal, genito-urinary and respiratory systems and commonly lead to neurological abnormalities. Skeletal involvement may be widespread leading to gross deformities including bony malformations of the orbit and, particularly, absence of the greater and lesser wings of the sphenoid. This latter may result in direct contact between the middle cranial fossa and orbit (spheno-orbital encephalocele) producing a characteristic pulsating proptosis with no bruit. Neurofibromata rarely undergo sarcomatous change.

Question 55

This 22-year-old man presented with a four-day history of pain, photophobia and slight blurring of vision. He had a history of similar episodes which had responded to treatment.

1. What is the diagnosis?
2. Name two associated systemic diseases.
3. What is the treatment of his ocular condition?

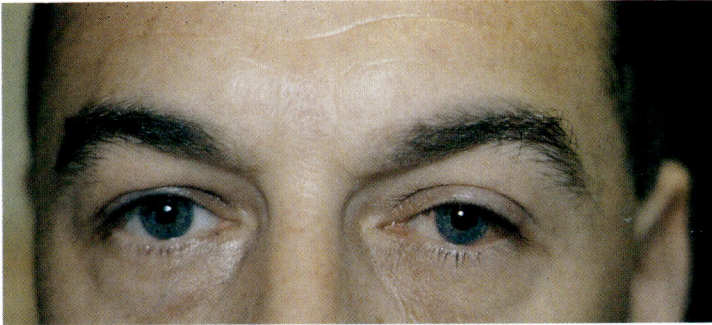

Answer to question 55

1. Acute iritis.
2. Ankylosing spondylitis, Reiter's syndrome, psoriatic arthritis, Behçet's disease, sarcoidosis, ulcerative colitis and Crohn's disease.
3. Topical steroids and atropine.

Acute anterior uveitis (iritis) typically presents with pain, photophobia, and redness with slight blurring of vision. Slit-lamp examination reveals cells in the anterior chamber and keratic precipitates (cellular deposits on the corneal endothelium). Posterior synechiae (adhesions between the pupillary margin and the anterior lens surface) develop easily and give rise to an irregular pupil. Treatment with steroids suppresses the inflammation, and dilatation of the pupil with atropine prevents the formation of posterior synechiae. In most cases no underlying cause can be found but a full medical history is essential. There are many causes of iritis but the common causes in a man of this age are listed above.

Question 56

This child developed a swelling of the right upper lid at the age of three months which has slowly increased in size since then.

1. What is the diagnosis?
2. Name one complication in this case.

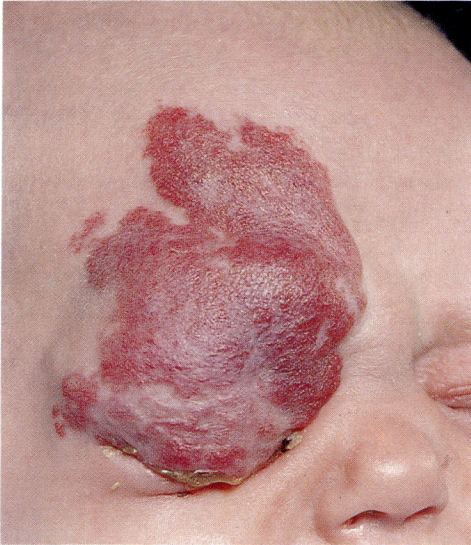

Answer to question 56

1. Capillary haemangioma (strawberry naevus).
2. Amblyopia.

This benign vascular tumour of childhood usually presents in the first three months of life, and may increase in size during the first year and then spontaneously regress and disappear by the age of six. It is more common in girls and typically increases in size with crying and straining. The tumour is most often situated in the anterior part of the orbit and involvement of the surrounding subcutaneous tissue gives the skin a dark red or blue discolouration.

Amblyopia (visual deprivation and anisometropic) may result, especially with larger upper lid tumours; rarely optic nerve compression or exposure keratopathy may result. Treatment is only indicated in those cases developing complications or those with a significant cosmetic defect. In such cases local steroid injection may be tried, often with dramatic results; such treatment must, however, be combined with correction of any astigmatism and treatment of amblyopia by occlusion of the good eye.

Question 57

This 62-year-old man has no ocular complaints.

1. What abnormality is shown?
2. What does it represent?
3. What tests would you perform in a young patient with this physical sign?

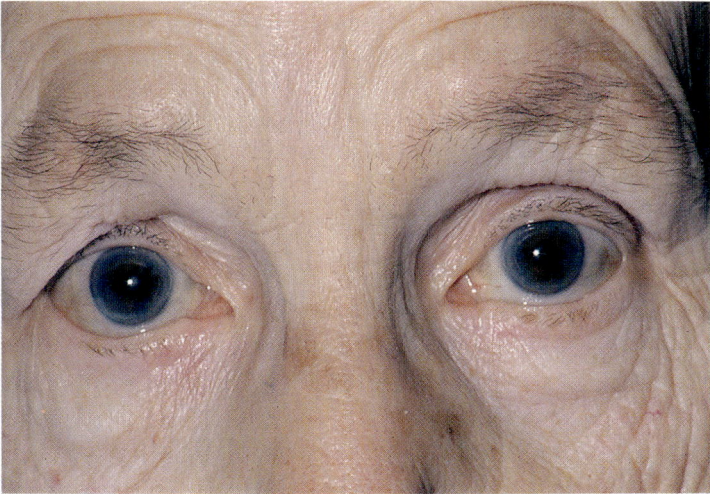

Answer to question 57

1. Arcus senilis.
2. Deposition of phospholipid and cholesterol in the corneal stroma.
3. Measurement of plasma lipids.

Arcus senilis is a normal phenomenon associated with ageing, but in patients under 50 it may be a manifestation of an underlying type II or III hyperlipidaemia (Frederickson's classification). In the former, arcus may be associated with eyelid xanthelasmata and in the latter with eruptive xanthomata. In both conditions lipaemia retinalis may develop when the plasma triglyceride level exceeds 2000 mg/ml.

Question 58

1. What abnormal physical sign is demonstrated?
2. What is the underlying disorder?
3. Name two associated systemic signs.

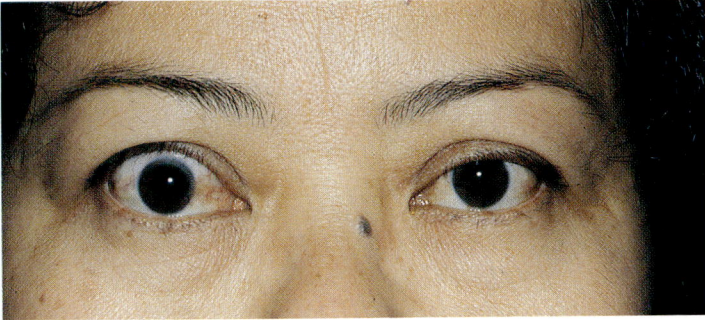

Answer to question 58

1. Right upper lid retraction.
2. Dysthyroid eye disease (Graves' ophthalmopathy).
3. Pretibial myxoedema and thyroid acropachy.

The eye signs associated with Graves' disease include lid retraction and lid lag which are pathognomonic, periorbital swelling, chemosis, prominent conjunctival vessels and limitation of ocular movements. Patients may be euthyroid, hyperthyroid or hypothyroid on presentation and thyroid antibodies are frequently present. Orbital CT scanning may show enlarged extraocular muscles, most commonly the medial and inferior rectus.

Upper lid retraction as in this case may result from overaction of Müller's muscle due to sympathetic overstimulation, overaction of the levator–superior rectus complex in response to contraction of the inferior rectus or infiltration of the levator palpebrae superioris. Mild cases may respond to topical guanethidine eye drops, but in more severe cases surgical correction is necessary and can produce good results providing the appearance has been stable for at least six months.

Question 59

This 67-year-old woman woke with a red eye.

What investigations should be performed?

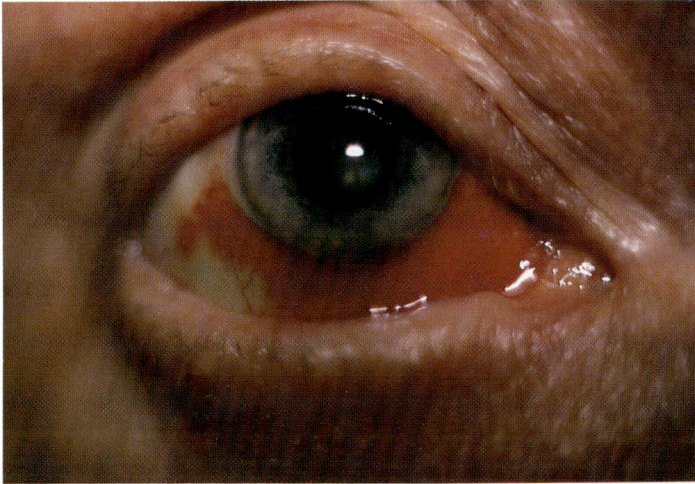

Answer to question 59

None.

An isolated subconjunctival haemorrhage in the absence of trauma is not associated with any ocular or systemic disease and no investigations are necessary. However, subconjunctival haemorrhage following trauma in which the posterior extent of the haemorrhage cannot be seen may indicate a fracture of the base of the skull.

Question 60

This patient was noted to have these fundal changes at a routine medical examination.

What is the diagnosis?

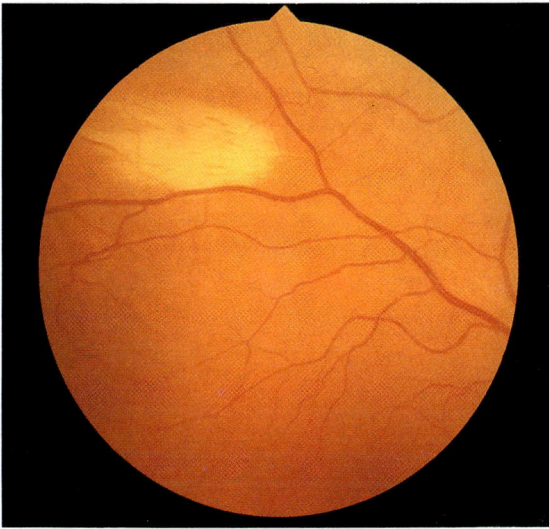

Answer to question 60

Myelinated nerve fibres.

Optic nerve myelination begins during the seventh month of gestation and is usually completed by about nine months. Myelination commences at the lateral geniculate body and spreads towards the eye, stopping at the lamina cribrosa. Occasionally myelination spreads onto the surface of the disc and may extend to involve the nerve fibre layer of the retina. Myelination at the disc may simulate disc oedema and myelinated fibres extend onto the retina as irregular feathery patches which may obscure the retinal vessels. The pattern of myelination is extremely variable and although seen most commonly next to the optic disc, peripheral patches of myelination may also occur. Regression of myelinated nerve fibres occurs with optic atrophy.

Question 61

1. What is the diagnosis?
2. What is the underlying systemic disease?
3. What is the management?

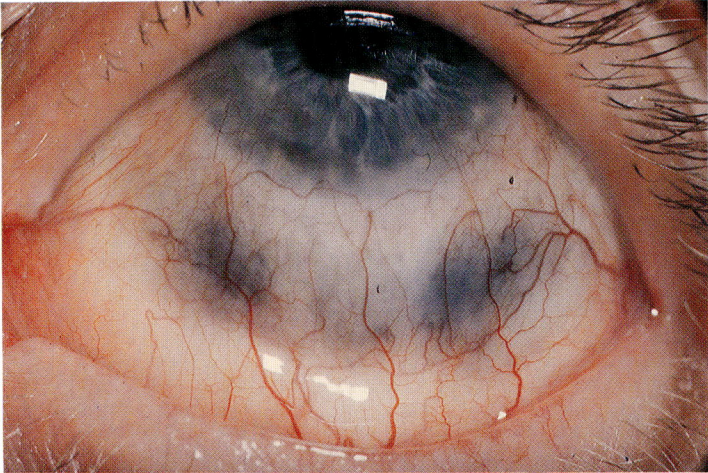

Answer to question 61

1. Scleromalacia perforans.
2. Rheumatoid arthritis.
3. Observation.

Scleromalacia perforans is found almost exclusively in elderly women with longstanding seropositive rheumatoid arthritis. An obliterative vasculitis leads to scleral thinning in the absence of ocular inflammation, and as the sclera becomes deficient large areas of uveal tissue become exposed. Scleral perforation is rare and no intervention is necessary.

Question 62

What is the diagnosis?

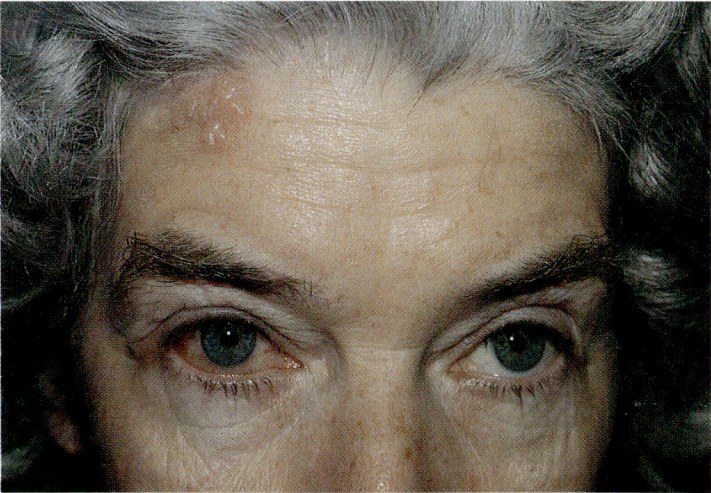

Answer to question 62

Herpes zoster ophthalmicus.

Herpes zoster is a common infection caused by the varicella zoster virus. It is thought that the virus lies dormant in a sensory ganglion, becomes reactivated and migrates down a sensory nerve to involve the skin. Seven to ten per cent of all cases of herpes zoster affect the ophthalmic division of the trigeminal nerve, and of these half will develop ocular involvement. The infection is most commonly seen in the elderly but can occur at any age, and may be seen in the acquired immunodeficiency syndrome. Ocular complications include: mucopurulent conjunctivitis, scleritis, keratitis, iritis and lid scarring leading to ptosis or ectropion. Neurological complications include: post-hepatic neuralgia, optic neuritis, cranial nerve palsies and rarely encephalitis.

Question 63

This 28-year-old man with severe asthma and eczema presented with gradual deterioration of vision.

1. What is the reason for his reduced vision?
2. What is the likely cause in this case?

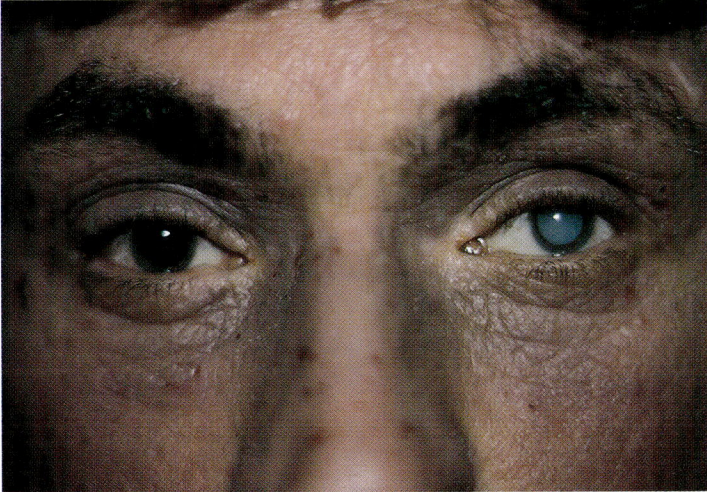

Answer to question 63

1. Cataract.
2. Long-term treatment with systemic steroids or an atopic cataract.

Cataracts may be associated with a wide variety of systemic diseases, the commonest of which include:

Chromosomal disorders
Down's syndrome.
Dystrophia myotonica.
Turner's syndrome.

Metabolic
Diabetes mellitus.
Galactosaemia.
Wilson's disease.
Hypocalcaemia.
Lowe's syndrome (amino aciduria).

Maternal infections
Rubella.
Cytomegalovirus.
Toxoplasmosis.

Atopic dermatitis

Systemic drugs
Corticosteroids.

Prolonged corticosteroid therapy whether topical or systemic is well known to be associated with the development of posterior subcapsular lens opacities. This type of cataract has a marked effect on vision and is associated with troublesome dazzle; the patient's vision is typically worse in bright sunlight, and when driving at night the effect on vision of oncoming car headlights may be likened to that of a dirty windscreen. There is no consistent relationship between the dose of steroids and the development of cataracts but it does seem that children are more susceptible than adults.

Question 64

1. What is the physical sign?
2. List three possible underlying medical conditions.

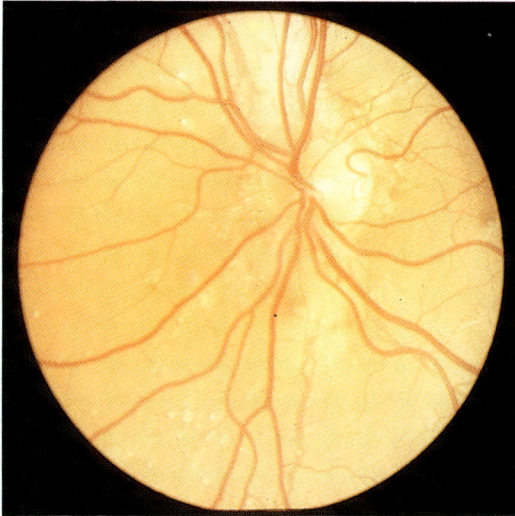

Answer to question 64

1. Angioid streaks.
2. (a) Pseudoxanthoma elasticum (see Question 36).
   (b) Ehlers–Danlos syndrome.
   (c) Sickle cell anaemia.
   (d) Paget's disease.

Angioid streaks are splits in Bruch's membrane; there is typically a peripapillary ring from which irregularly radiating streaks extend towards the periphery. Angioid streaks are usually asymptomatic but visual symptoms may occur with the development of subretinal neovascularisation in the papillomacular region. This is seen on fluorescein angiography and the affected areas may be amenable to laser therapy. Angioid streaks may occur as an isolated finding or in association with any of the above conditions.

Question 65

This 62-year-old patient complained of constant and severe ocular pain which kept her awake at night.

1. What is the underlying systemic abnormality?
2. What is the most likely cause of her ocular pain?

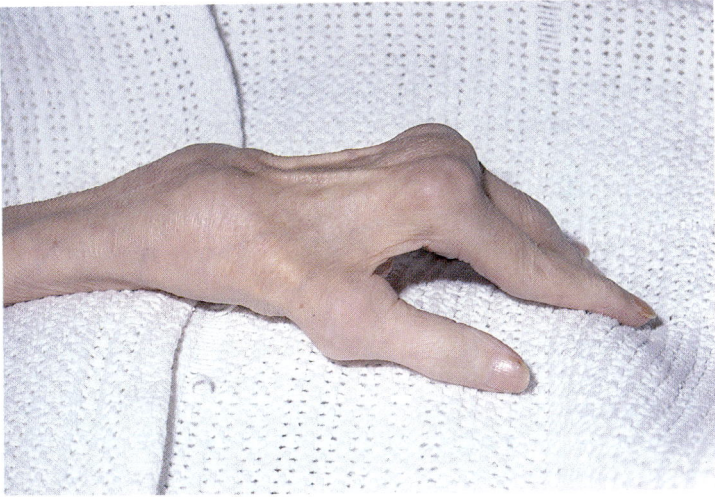

Answer to question 65

1. Rheumatoid arthritis.
2. Scleritis.

This patient has the characteristic signs of rheumatoid arthritis. The ocular complications of adult rheumatoid arthritis are most commonly seen in patients with extra-articular manifestations of the disease. Keratoconjunctivitis sicca is the commonest manifestation of the disease and may be associated with a dry mouth (xerostomia). Patients complain of grittiness and burning in the eyes and obtain symptomatic relief from artificial tear preparations. Scleritis is seen in 0.5% of patients with rheumatoid arthritis and presents with severe ocular pain that typically disturbs sleep, and the eye is injected with a bluish discolouration. It is a potentially sight-threatening condition which may require treatment with systemic steroids and immunosuppressants. Episcleritis may also occur but is a benign condition responding to topical treatment. Rarely a keratitis may be seen leading to corneal melting. Asymptomatic scleral thinning without inflammation may occur leading to scleromalacia perforans. Iatrogenic ocular problems can develop with prolonged use of steroids leading to posterior subcapsular cataracts, and anti-malarials may produce a retinopathy.

Iritis is rare in adult rheumatoid arthritis, but a chronic iridocyclitis is seen in the pauci-articular form of juvenile rheumatoid arthritis. The iritis is asymptomatic and can be complicated by cataracts, glaucoma and band keratopathy; it is therefore important that patients at risk are examined regularly by slit-lamp biomicroscopy. The iritis is bilateral in 70% of cases and about half the affected patients are HLA-DW5 positive.

Question 66

What is the diagnosis?

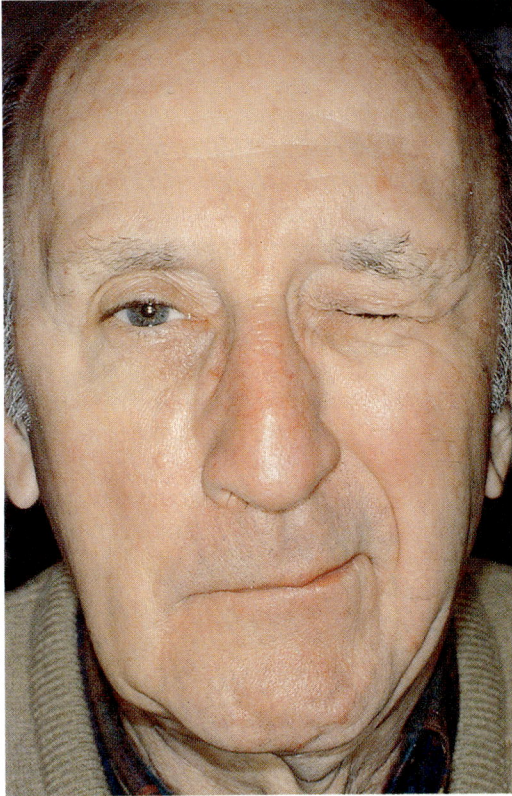

Answer to question 66

Hemifacial spasm.

Hemifacial spasm is characterised by intermittent unilateral facial twitching which initially involves the orbicularis oculi and spreads over a period of time to involve the whole face. The rhythmical contractions may last only seconds or continue for hours, and such prolonged contractions may lead to cosmetically disfiguring grimacing with eyelid closure. The condition is exacerbated by stress, and in contrast to blepharospasm may occur during sleep.

Hemifacial spasm is thought to be due to compression of the facial nerve by a tortuous anterior or posterior inferior cerebellar artery, but in all cases a structural posterior fossa lesion should be excluded radiologically. Initial treatment is with repeated injections of botulinum toxin, which is most effective when the contractions are localised to the orbicularis region. In severe cases a large percentage of patients will respond to surgery with placement of a sponge between the artery and the nerve, but facial paralysis and ipsilateral hearing loss may result.

The condition must be distinguished from essential blepharospasm, focal cortical seizures and facial myokymia.

Question 67

A 57-year-old woman noticed reduced vision in the right eye on waking. On examination her right visual acuity was 6/24, a right afferent pupillary defect was noted and the visual field is shown.

1. What is the diagnosis?
2. What one investigation would you perform?

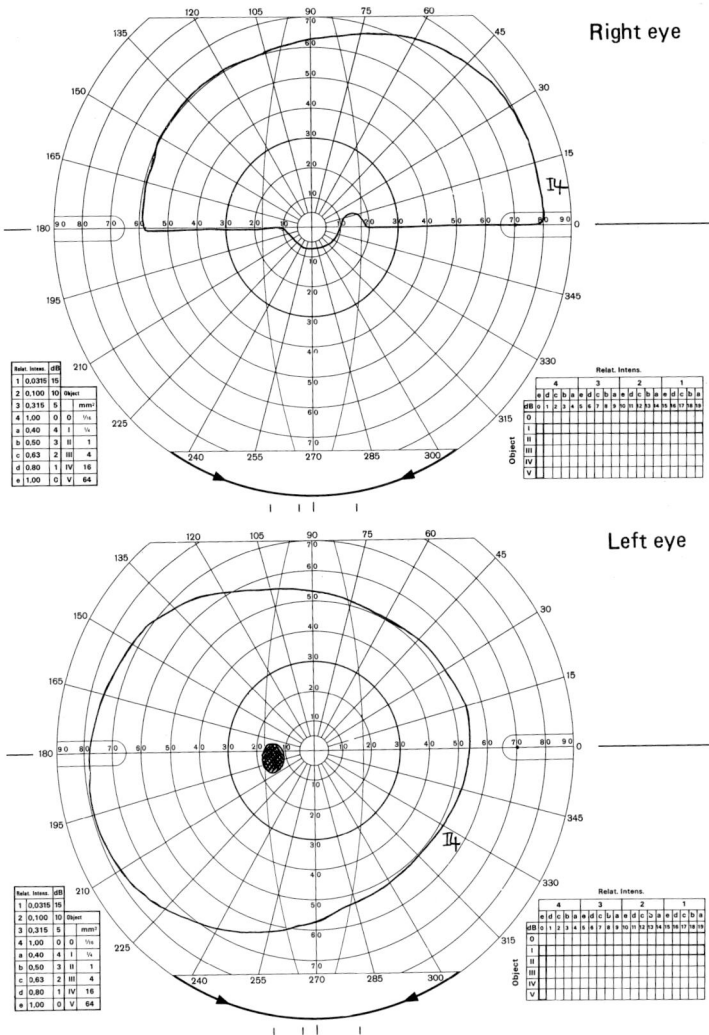

Right eye

Left eye

Answer to question 67

1. Anterior ischaemic optic neuropathy (non-arteritic).
2. Erythrocyte sedimentation rate.

Anterior ischaemic optic neuropathy (AION) is characterised by sudden loss of vision, optic disc swelling, an afferent pupillary defect and visual field defects. Non-arteritic AION must be differentiated from that associated with giant cell arteritis. Affected patients are usually between 45 and 65 years old and may have a history of diabetes mellitus, hypertension or cardiovascular disease, but are often in good health. Visual loss is typically sudden and painless; vision sometimes deteriorates over a few days due to oedematous compression of remaining viable nerve fibres. The superior hemisphere of the disc is most commonly affected producing the characteristic inferior altitudinal field defect. Improvement in vision is rare due to the subsequent development of optic atrophy. In the acute phase the disc swelling may be diffuse or sectorial and peripapillary haemorrhages are common. The oedema usually resolves over 1–2 months and the involved portion of the disc becomes atrophic. In addition optic discs may appear small in size. There is no effective treatment but it is important to control any underlying hypertension or diabetes mellitus.

In 25% of patients AION develops in the fellow eye months to years later and produces a pseudo Foster–Kennedy syndrome with disc oedema in one eye and optic atrophy in the other.

Question 68

This patient with a history of severe head injury presented with a painful eye and diplopia.

1. What is the diagnosis?
2. List three clinical signs associated with this condition.

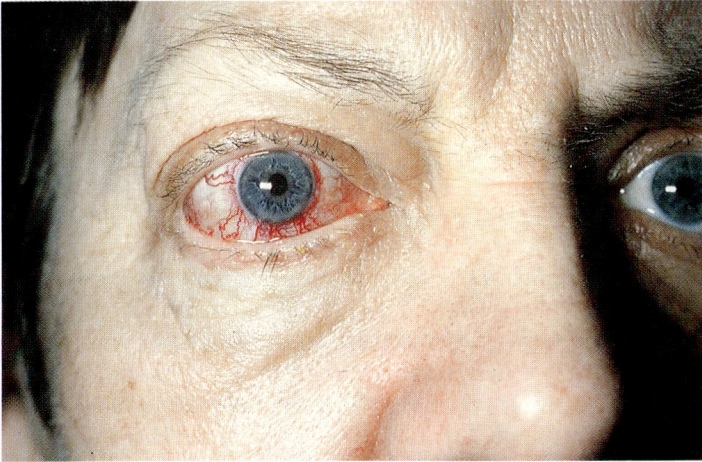

Answer to question 68

1. Carotico-cavernous fistula.
2. The following clinical signs may be present:
   (a) third, fourth, and sixth cranial nerve palsies (the sixth is the most commonly affected).
   (b) pulsating exophthalmos.
   (c) ocular bruit.
   (d) arterialisation of conjunctival vessels and chemosis.
   (e) congestion of retinal vessels, disc swelling and haemorrhage.
   (f) visual loss from glaucoma or retinal ischaemia.

Carotico-cavernous fistulae are most commonly (>75%) the consequence of head injury, usually frontal and ipsilateral relative to the lesion. The wall of the carotid artery or one of its branches ruptures into the cavernous sinus, resulting in an arterio-venous fistula with a high flow rate. Fistulae with lower flow rates may occur following spontaneous rupture of branches of the external carotid artery in the dura, thus producing a communication with the dural veins draining into the cavernous sinus. Such dural fistulae are seen most commonly in middle-aged women and in 50% of cases respond spontaneously.

The clinical presentation of arterio-venous fistulae depends on the rapidity of onset, the extent of vascular shunting, the increase in orbital venous pressure and consequent orbital or ocular hypoxia. In carotico-cavernous fistulae CT scan reveals dilatation of the superior ophthalmic vein and the diagnosis is confirmed by carotid angiography. Fistulae may be treated by embolisation with a balloon catheter via the internal carotid artery or superior ophthalmic vein. Glaucoma may be difficult to control in those cases, responding poorly to topical medical therapy and surgical drainage procedures.

Question 69

1. What is the diagnosis?
2. What neurological disorder is associated?

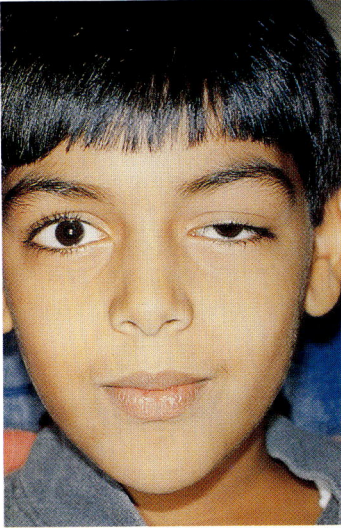

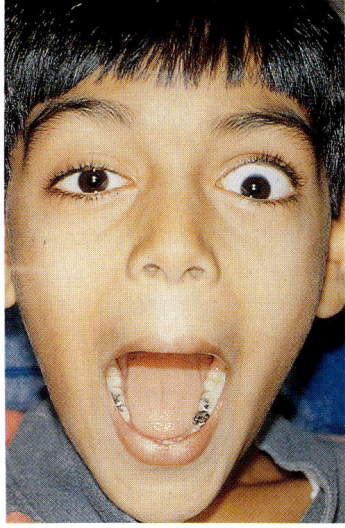

Answer to question 69

1. Marcus Gunn jaw winking ptosis.
2. None.

Marcus Gunn jaw winking ptosis is characterised by reduction of the ptosis on opening the mouth or moving the jaw to one side, usually the opposite side from the ptosis. It is always congenital and usually unilateral. The abnormal synkinesis between the pterygoid muscles and levator palpebrae superioris muscle, which is thought to account for the jaw wink, is probably the result of a developmental brainstem abnormality. The patient may present with either the ptosis or the jaw wink as the main symptom and the surgical technique differs in each. Synkinetic movements of the eyelid associated with ptosis are also seen with aberrant regeneration of the III nerve.

Question 70

This is a fundal photograph of a 6-month-old baby who had developed grand mal fits whilst in the care of a babysitter.

1. What is the diagnosis?
2. What investigation should be performed?

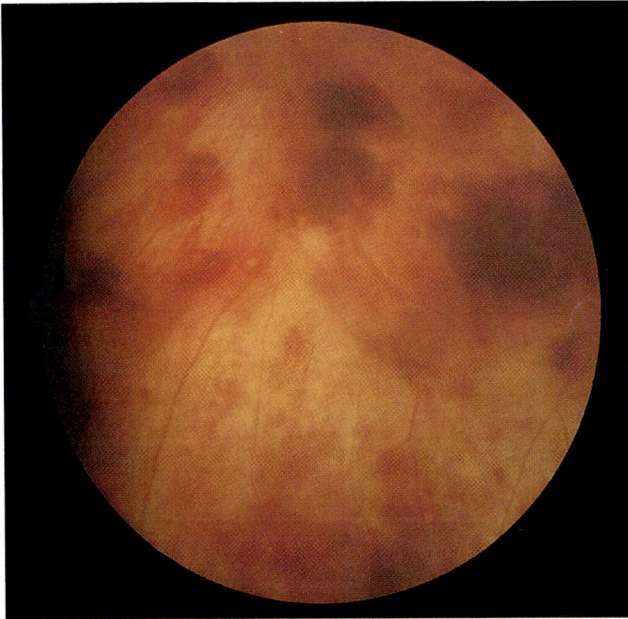

Answer to question 70

1. Non-accidental injury.
2. Cerebral CT Scan.

Most cases of NAI in children occur before the age of 3 years and ocular involvement is common. Retinal haemorrhages may arise from direct head trauma, follow thoracic or abdominal compression or be associated with 'the shaken baby syndrome' in which shearing forces from shaking the infant cause mechanical damage to the ocular and cerebral vasculature. The intraocular haemorrhages may be retinal, pre-retinal and vitreal. Although many cases heal without complication they may lead to optic atrophy, macular scarring or retinal detachment. Other ophthalmic manifestations of NAI include periorbital swelling and bruising, subconjunctival haemorrhages, hyphaemas, cataract and dislocated lenses. As intraocular haemorrhages are frequently associated with intracranial haemorrhages and subdural haematomas, all patients should have a cerebral CT scan even in the absence of head trauma or neurological signs.

Question 71

1. What is the diagnosis?
2. List three ocular features of this condition.
3. How may clinical examination confirm the diagnosis?

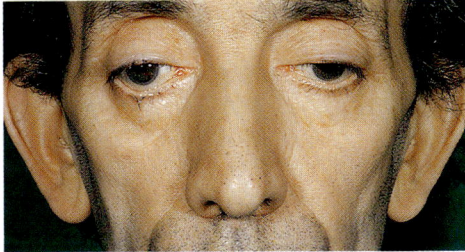

142

Answer to question 71

1. Dystrophia myotonica.
2. (a) Cataracts.
   (b) Ptosis.
   (c) External ophthalmoplegia.
   (d) Pigmentary retinopathy.
3. Demonstration of myotonia.

Dystrophia myotonica is usually inherited as an autosomal dominant condition with variable penetrance. The clinical features become more pronounced in successive generations and the presence of cataracts in a previous generation may be the only evidence of the disease. Characteristically, there is an early appearance of polychromatic glistening granules in the subcapsular and cortical areas of the lens which progress to a posterior subcapsular cataract. Both sexes are affected and may present at any age with myotonia and weakness but onset is usually between 20 and 50 years of age. The other characteristic features include: facial myopathy, particularly wasting of the temporalis muscles; distal muscular atrophy and myopathy of respiratory muscles; frontal baldness; gonadal atrophy and infertility; cardiomyopathy; frequent infections due to immunoglobulin abnormalities; poor gastric motility; low IQ and dementia.

The diagnosis is made on clinical features and EMG. In some cases, the myotonia is improved by procainamide or phenytoin.

Question 72

This young man complained of mild discomfort of the left eye.

What is the diagnosis?

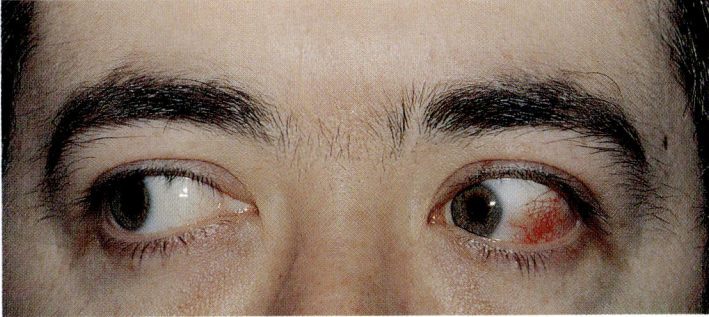

Answer to question 72

Episcleritis.

Episcleritis is a common, benign, self-limiting inflammation of the episclera which may be bilateral, occurring principally in young adults. Episcleritis may be nodular or diffuse, but the nodules are mobile on the underlying sclera. It is important to distinguish episcleritis from scleritis, which is a destructive vasculitis of the vessels of the anterior chambers of the eye. The latter is more commonly associated with rheumatoid arthritis, SLE, Wegener's granulomatosis, polyarteritis nodosa and Crohn's disease. The principal symptoms of episcleritis, namely mild discomfort and watering of the eye, are mild in comparison to the severe pain, photophobia and visual disturbance of scleritis.

Question 73

This patient is sitting in a dimly lit room.

1. What physical sign is shown?
2. List three possible causes.

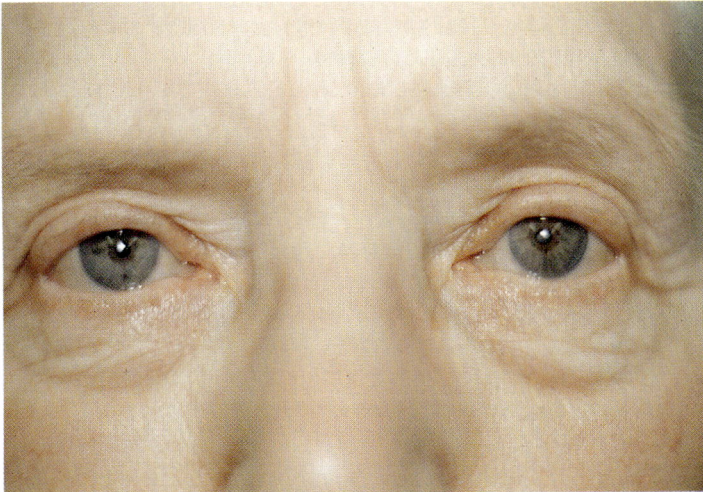

Answer to question 73

1. Bilateral miosis.
2. The diagnosis includes:
   (a) drug-induced — topical administration (e.g. pilocarpine) or systemic medications such as morphine or barbiturates.
   (b) pontine lesion.
   (c) Argyll Robertson pupils (more usually irregular or pseudo Argyll Robertson pupils as in diabetes).
   (d) bilateral Horner's syndrome.
   (e) posterior synechia — iritis.

Interruption of the sympathetic fibres, either centrally or peripherally, results in miosis due to paralysis of the pupillary dilator muscles. The sympathetic nerve endings of the iris may also be affected by topical administration of certain drugs. The pupillary dilator sympathetic fibres arise in the posterior part of the hypothalamus, pass through the lateral tegmentum of the midbrain, pons, medulla and spinal cord to the level of T1–2, where they synapse with the lateral horn cells, giving rise to preganglionic fibres which travel to the superior cervical ganglion via the stellate ganglion where they synapse. The post-ganglionic fibres pass along the internal carotid arteries through the cavernous sinus to join the first division of the trigeminal nerve, reaching the eye as the long ciliary nerve.

Question 74

1. What abnormality is shown?
2. Name two possible causes.

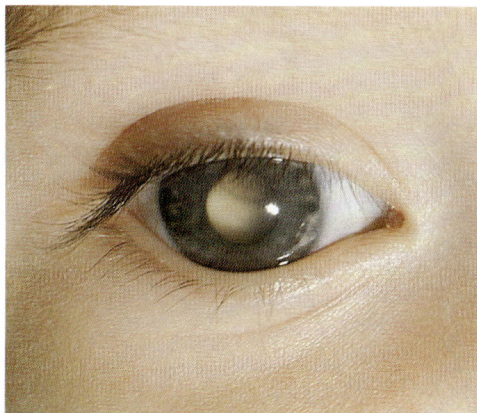

Answer to question 74

1. Leucocoria (white pupil).
2. Congenital cataract, retinoblastoma, persistent primary hyperplastic vitreous, coloboma of the retina, retinopathy of prematurity, toxocara endophthalmitis, Coats' disease, intraocular foreign body and rare retinal dysplasias.

All children with leucocoria should be urgently referred to an opthalmologist. A careful clinical history including a genetic and neonatal history followed by examination under a general anaesthetic will provide the diagnosis in the vast majority of cases. The treatment depends on the underlying cause.

Question 75

1. What field defect is shown?
2. What is the investigation of choice?

Right eye

Left eye

Answer to question 75

1. Bitemporal hemianopia.
2. CT scanning of the optic chiasm.

Lesions of the optic chiasm produce temporal visual field loss in both eyes that typically do not cross the midline. If the central visual fibres are involved reduced visual acuity and colour vision with a central scotoma may be seen. An afferent pupillary defect may be present if the involvement is asymmetrical and optic disc pallor may occur in longstanding cases.

A compressive lesion is the usual cause of a chiasmal syndrome, most commonly a pituitary tumour: other less common causes include craniopharyngioma, meningioma, glioma and suprasellar aneurysm. Demyelination and trauma are rare causes.

Lesions which may mimic a bitemporal hemianopia include tilted optic discs, nasal sector retinitis pigmentosa, bilateral centrocaecal scotomas, papilloedema with greatly enlarged blind spots, and redundant overhanging lid tissue. An important clinical point is that in these conditions the field defect does not extend exactly to the vertical meridian as it does in chiasmal lesions.

Question 76

1. What is the diagnosis?
2. List four underlying causes.
3. What blood tests would you perform?

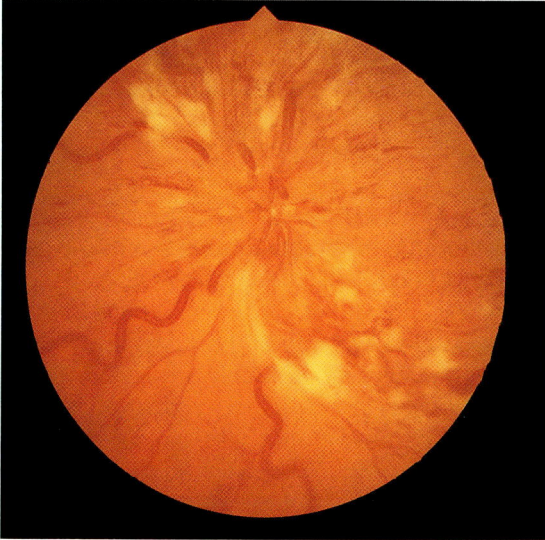

Answer to question 76

1. Central retinal vein occlusion.
2. (a) Chronic open-angle glaucoma.
   (b) Vascular disease, i.e. retinal periphlebitis which may be seen in sarcoidosis and Behçet's syndrome.
   (c) Venous stasis retinopathy, blood dyscrasias, Waldenstrom's macroglobulinaemia, multiple myeloma, polycythaemia rubra vera.
   (d) Benign central retinal vasculitis.
3. Full blood count, blood film, ESR, protein electrophoresis.

Central retinal vein occlusions (CRVO) typically present in elderly patients with a moderate to severe reduction in visual acuity which is painless and of rapid onset. Examination reveals a grossly haemorrhagic fundus, marked venous dilatation, cotton wool spots and swelling of the optic disc. Occasionally, the symptoms are very mild and only a few retinal haemorrhages appear. In longstanding cases venous collateral vessels may be seen on the optic disc, which are thought to shunt blood from the retinal circulation to the lower pressure choroidal plexus draining into the vortex veins. Fluorescein angiography shows venous and capillary leakage at the optic disc and in the retina with macular oedema. In some cases symptoms improve over 2–3 months as the central retinal veins recanalise or collateral vessels develop. In severe cases macular oedema persists or rubeosis iridis develops progressing to thrombotic glaucoma with consequent visual loss.

Question 77

This child was referred by her general practitioner because of a difference in the colour of her irides.

1. What is the diagnosis?
2. Name one other cause of heterochromia.

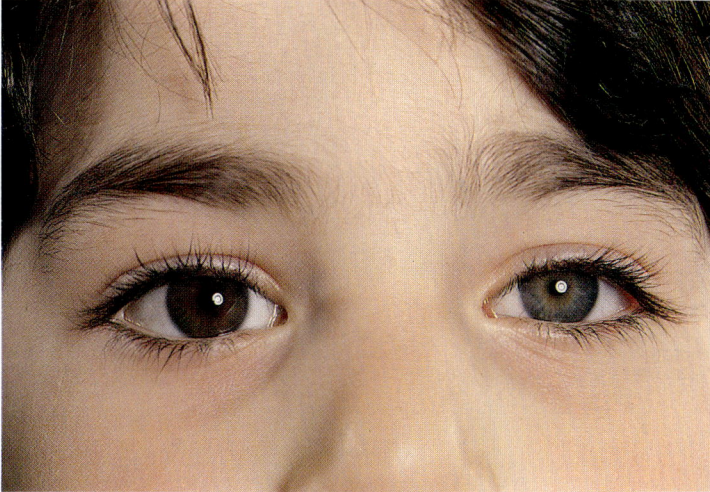

Answer to question 77

1. Congenital left Horner's syndrome.
2. (a) Congenital: Simple idiopathic.
   (b) Acquired: Fuch's heterochromic cyclitis.
       Iris atrophy following trauma or inflammation.
       Ocular siderosis: iron deposition from a retained intraocular foreign body.
       Iris melanoma.

Question 78

1. What is the diagnosis?
2. How may this condition affect the eyes?

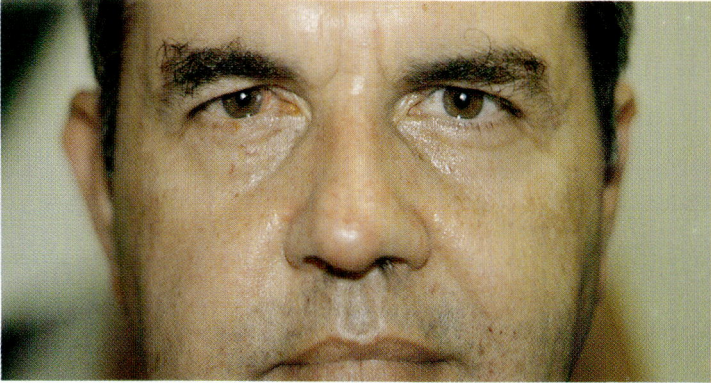

Answer to question 78

1. Acne rosacea.
2. Chronic blepharitis and keratitis.

Acne rosacea is a chronic facial dermatitis principally affecting fair-skinned people and more commonly seen in women. It is characterised by cutaneous telangiectasis, facial papules and pustules, diffuse erythema and sebaceous gland hypertrophy. The lesions are distributed principally on the cheeks, nose, forehead and chin. Rhinophyma is the most advanced form of the disease. The cause is unknown. Ocular involvement is common and variable in severity. Marginal blepharitis, meibomionitis and conjunctival hyperaemia are seen frequently. Keratitis is also a feature with recurrent marginal infiltrates, corneal thinning and vascularisation, principally in the inferotemporal and inferonasal quadrants. Systemic tetracycline and erythromycin help both the ocular and skin manifestations. Topical tetracycline may be used on the skin and topical corticosteroids are an effective short-term measure in controlling the blepharoconjunctivitis and keratitis.

Question 79

1. What is the investigation?
2. What does it show?
3. List three common presenting symptoms.

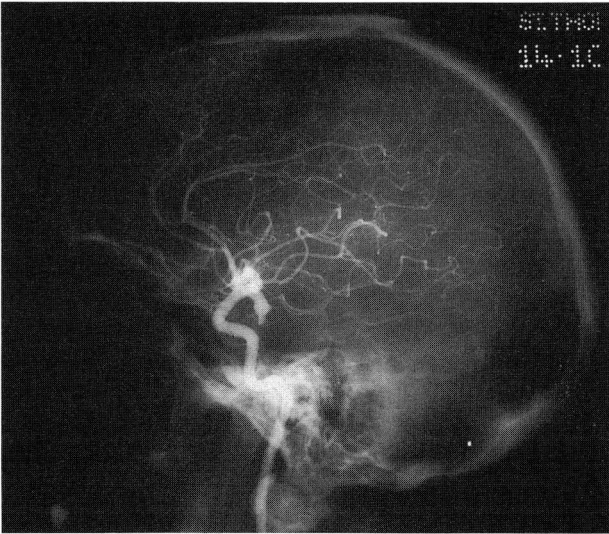

Answer to question 79

1. Cerebral angiogram.
2. An aneurysm of the posterior communicating artery.
3. (a) Sudden severe ipsilateral headache.
    (b) Supraorbital pain.
    (c) Diplopia.

Acute presentation of a painful isolated third nerve palsy in adults is most commonly due to diabetic vascular disease or compression of the third nerve by an arterial aneurysm. The latter should always be suspected if there is pupillary involvement. Carotid angiography should be performed prior to surgical ligation of the aneurysm.

Question 80

This 20-year-old woman presented with a five-day history of blurring of vision in her right eye.

1. What is the likely diagnosis?
2. Name an associated clinical feature.
3. How would you confirm the diagnosis?

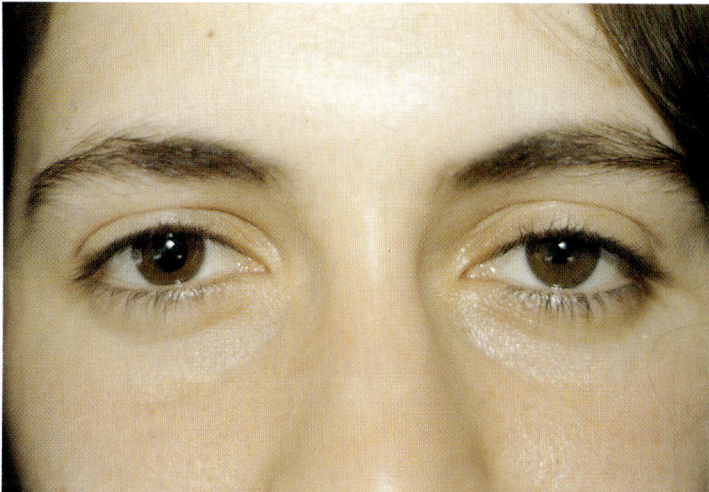

Answer to question 80

1. Holmes–Adie pupil.
2. Depressed deep tendon reflexes.
3. Hypersensitivity of the pupil to 0.125% pilocarpine or 2.5% methylcholine which do not constrict a normal pupil.

Holmes–Adie pupil is an idiopathic benign lesion at the ciliary ganglion or post-ganglionic neurone, most commonly seen in young women. Although unilateral in 80% of cases there is a tendency for the other eye to become involved later. Typically the onset is abrupt with paralysis of accommodation being the main symptom. The dilated pupil shows a sluggish response to light, but may constrict after prolonged exposure. The near response may be brisk. Vermiform movements of the iris may be seen on slit-lamp examination. With time accommodation recovers and the pupil becomes smaller. Denervation hypersensitivity may be demonstrated by weak cholinergic agents.

This condition should be distinguished from pharmacological mydriasis of the pupil, e.g. by atropine, in which case there would be no constriction of the pupil to light, accommodation or normal strength cholinergics, e.g. pilocarpine 4%.

Question 81

What is the diagnosis?

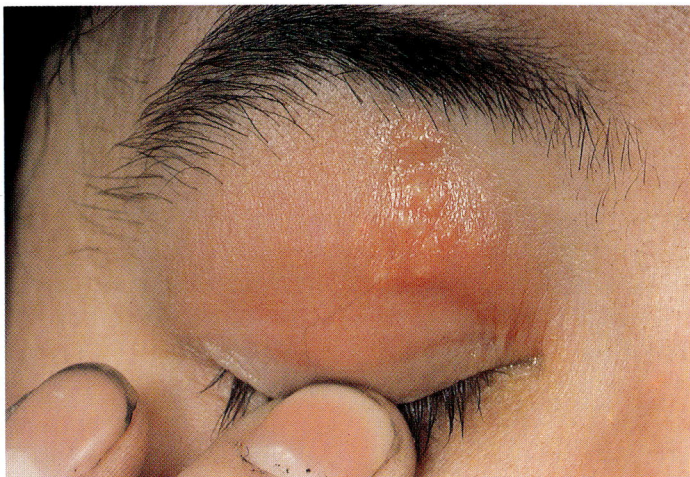

Answer to question 81

Herpes simplex.

Primary infection with herpes simplex occurs in non-immune subjects and is usually acquired in early life. The disease may be subclinical or be associated with fever and malaise. Skin lesions may involve the lids and periorbital area and begin as vescicles which ulcerate, crust and heal without scarring. These skin lesions may be associated with a follicular conjunctivitis, mild keratitis and pre-auricular lymphadenopathy. Unlike primary infection, recurrent herpes simplex is not associated with systemic features and commonly involves the cornea producing the classical dendritic ulcer. Untreated this may progress to corneal scarring and vascularisation.

Question 82

This 30-year-old man complained of diplopia.

1. What is the diagnosis?
2. List two possible causes.

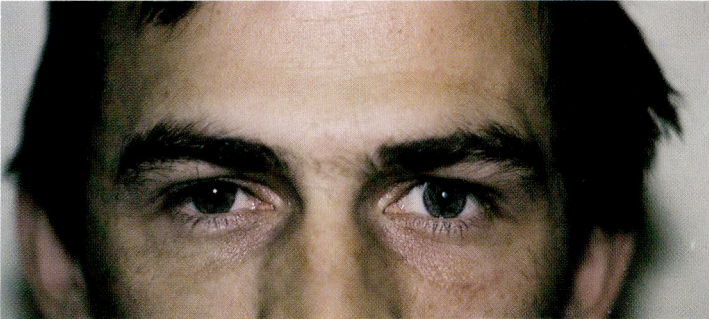

A Patient looking straight ahead.

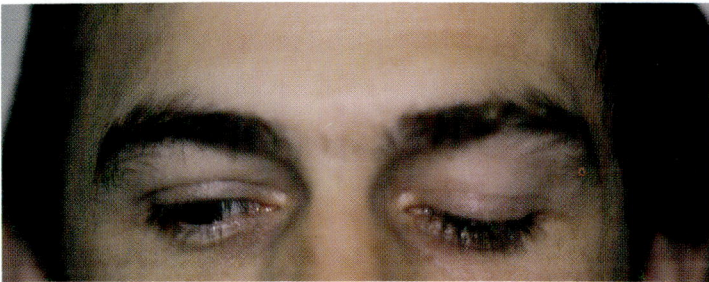

B Patient looking down.

Answer to question 82

1. Aberrant regeneration of the third cranial nerve (right).
2. (a) Trauma.
   (b) Compressive lesions of the third cranial nerve, e.g.
   posterior communicating artery aneurysm or
   meningioma.

Aberrant regeneration most commonly follows traumatic third
nerve palsies associated with severe head injuries, developing
most commonly 8–12 weeks after trauma. It can also be seen
following longstanding compression of the nerve, but is not a
feature of ischaemic lesions of the nerve. The mechanism for
the aberrant movements is not known but it is thought to be of
supranuclear origin rather than a peripheral misdirection of
axons. The signs suggestive of aberrant regeneration are:
1. Elevation of the upper eyelid on downgaze (pseudo-Graefe
   phenomenon) and on adduction.
2. Adduction or retraction of the globe on attempted upgaze or
   downgaze.
3. Pupillary constriction on attempted adduction with sluggish
   response to light (light-near dissociation).

Question 83

This patient has no ocular complaint.

1. What is the abnormal physical sign?
2. What is the most likely diagnosis?

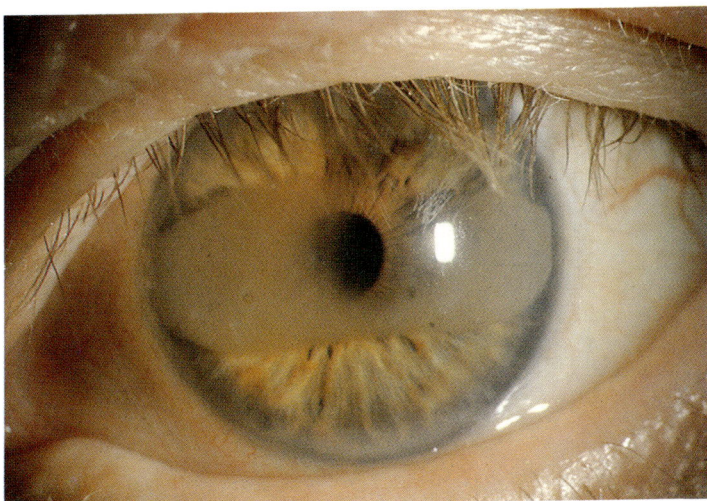

Answer to question 83

1. Band keratopathy.
2. Hyperparathyroidism.

Band keratopathy is seen in hypercalcaemia, as a sequel to almost any severe ocular disease, or may be idiopathic. Calcium is deposited in the superficial stroma in the Bowman's layer and in the deep epithelium, and the distribution is characteristically interpalpebral with a clear zone between the edge of the band and the limbus. Prolonged hypercalcaemia may also result in conjunctival crystals outside the limbus or under the eyelids.

Question 84

1. What is the diagnosis?
2. What abnormalities are shown?
3. List three conditions associated with this retinal abnormality.

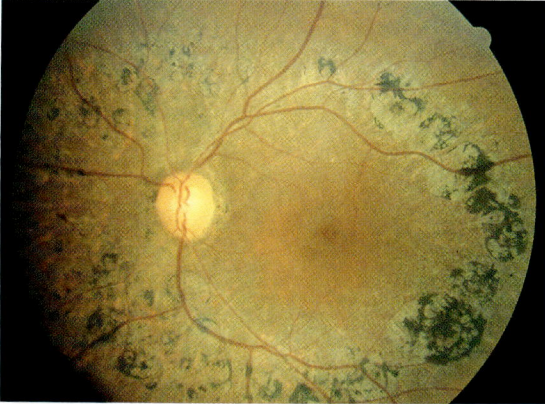

Answer to question 84

1. Retinitis pigmentosa.
2. (a) Bone spicule pigmentation.
   (b) Optic disc pallor.
   (c) Attenuated retinal vessels.
3. Associated conditions include: Friedreich's ataxia, Laurence–Moon–Biedl syndrome, Refsum's disease, chronic progressive external ophthalmoplegia, Usher's syndrome, abetalipoproteinaemia.

Retinitis pigmentosa describes a group of conditions characterised by night blindness, visual field constriction and the typical fundus appearance. The disease affects the photoreceptor:retinal pigment epithelium complex, predominantly affecting rods. Males are affected more frequently than females (3:1) and inheritance is either dominant, recessive or sex-linked. The perimacular zones are affected first, causing a partial or complete ring scotoma. As the disease progresses peripheral constriction of the visual fields occurs until the patient is totally blind apart from a small central tubular field of vision. This persists as the pigmentary degeneration spares the fovea. Photophobia and glare are important secondary symptoms. No treatment has been found to alter the rate of progression and management is aimed at educating the patient in the early stages of the disease and genetic counselling. Cataract formation often exacerbates the visual disability.

The electroretinogram response is lost early in the disease, sometimes before fundal changes are noted. Sectoral retinitis pigmentosa is a variant of the disease in which only one small area of the retina is involved in each eye.

Systemic diseases should be excluded in all patients, particularly potentially treatable disorders such as Refsum's disease and abetalipoproteinaemia.

Question 85

This child was noted by the optician to have reduced abduction of the left eye at routine examination: she was asymptomatic.

What is the diagnosis?

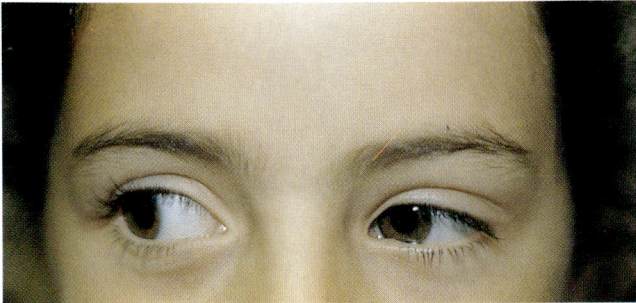

A

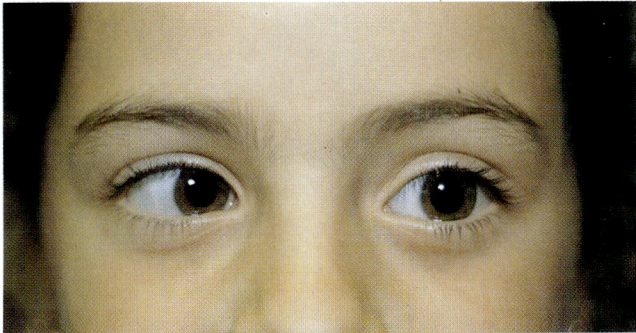

B

Answer to question 85

Duane's retraction syndrome.

This child has Duane's retraction syndrome, the characteristic features of which include: limitation of abduction, normal or slightly defective adduction, retraction of the globe on adduction with narrowing of the palpebral fissure and a face turned to the affected side. The eyes are usually straight in the primary position with binocular function, although a convergent squint is present in some cases. The condition may be unilateral, most commonly affecting the left eye, or bilateral. Most patients with Duane's syndrome are asymptomatic and surgery is rarely indicated.

The aetiology of Duane's syndrome is uncertain but thought to be the result of paradoxical innervation of the medial and lateral recti.

The main differential diagnosis is a VI cranial nerve palsy in which there is reduced abduction with a large-angle esotropia. Rare causes of reduced abduction in a child include Moebius' syndrome (bilateral VI and VII cranial nerve palsies), strabismus fixus, nystagmus blockage syndrome and oculomotor apraxia (congenital paralysis of saccadic eye movements).

Question 86

This patient with renal failure was complaining of watery eyes.

What is the diagnosis?

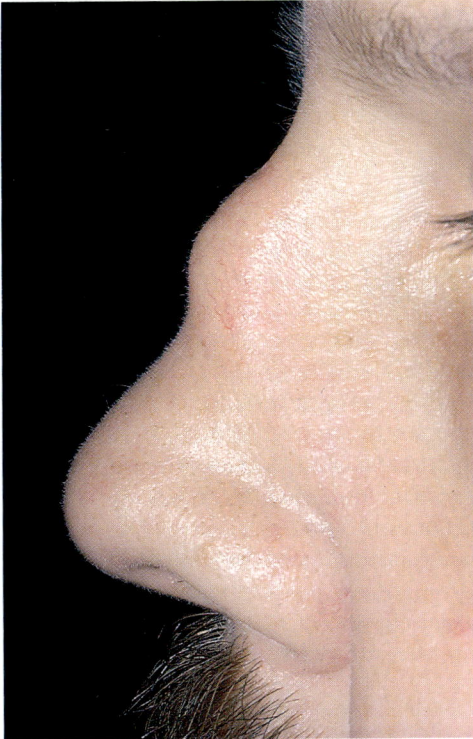

Answer to question 86

Wegener's granulomatosis.

Wegener's granulomatosis is a diffuse systemic disease. Characteristic features consist of granulomas and vasculitis of upper and lower respiratory tracts, focal necrotising glomerulonephritis and generalised small vessel vasculitis. Nasal and sinus symptoms are the most common presenting features with nasal obstruction and a serosanguinous discharge: late in the course of the disease septal perforations and severe nasal saddling are seen. Severe constitutional symptoms are common, e.g. fever, malaise, weight loss and night sweats. Pulmonary involvement is common and renal disease with rapidly progressive renal failure is the primary cause of death. The disease may also involve the middle ear, skin, joints, heart and central nervous system.

Ocular manifestations are seen in approximately 40% of patients, most frequently secondary to contiguous granulomatous sinus or nasal disease. Patients present with proptosis, obstruction of the nasolacrimal ducts or optic nerve compression. Other features include scleritis, keratitis, retinal vasculitis, and cranial nerve palsies.

The diagnosis is confirmed histologically by the presence of necrotising granulomas and vasculitis in the biopsy specimen, usually nasal mucosa. Cyclophosphamide is the treatment of choice and corticosteroids also have a role.

Question 87

This patient complained of diplopia when looking down.

What is the diagnosis?

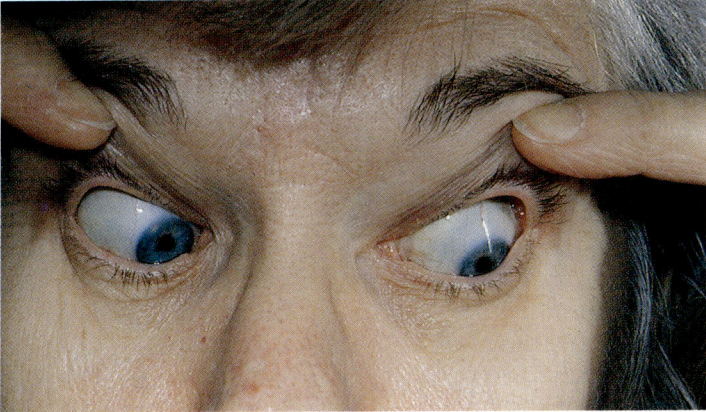

Answer to question 87

Right IV nerve palsy.

Patients with IV nerve palsies usually present with vertical diplopia, particularly in downgaze and frequently adopt a head posture with the head tilted and turned away from the affected side. On examination of the extraocular movements there is limitation of downgaze in adduction in the affected eye. The Bielschowsky head tilt test will help confirm the diagnosis.

The commonest cause of an acquired IV nerve palsy is closed head trauma; only rarely are microvascular episodes or neoplasms responsible. Congenital IV nerve palsy is common, but may not present until adult life as a result of breakdown of fusional mechanisms; in these cases the patients often have an abnormal head posture which may be apparent on old photographs and provide a clue to the diagnosis.

Bilateral IV nerve palsies are invariably the result of severe blunt head trauma. The main symptom is of torsional diplopia, which may be severe. Asymmetry is common and all traumatic cases should be suspected as being bilateral. Ocular muscle surgery is indicated in patients with troublesome symptoms.

Question 88

This 67-year-old man complained of chronically sore eyes and difficulty in swallowing. Conjunctival biopsy demonstrated deposition of immunoglobulin and complement in the basement membrane by direct immunofluorescence.

What is the diagnosis?

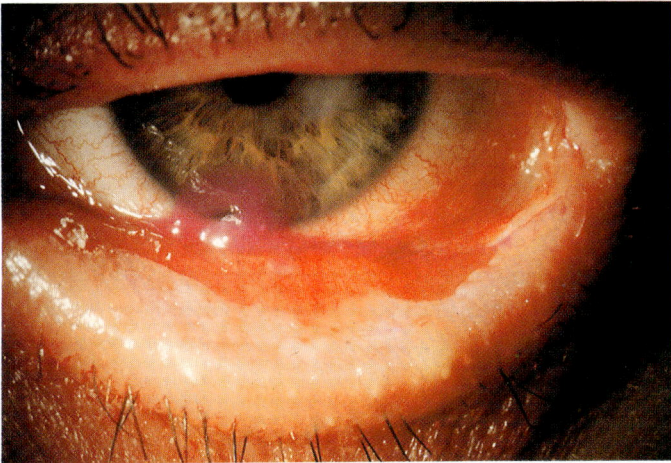

Answer to question 88

Ocular cicatricial pemphigoid (benign mucous membrane pemphigoid).

Pemphigoid is a rare autoimmune disorder which may involve skin and oesophageal, buccal, laryngeal, conjunctival and orogenital mucosae. The majority of patients presenting with classical bullous pemphigoid are over 60 years. Skin lesions predominate and tense thick-walled blisters develop: mucosal lesions are largely confined to the mouth. In contrast to this, ocular cicatricial pemphigoid is rarely associated with skin lesions and occurs in a younger age group, usually affecting patients over 45 years. Conjunctival involvement usually begins insidiously as a non-specific conjunctivitis which progresses to scarring and obliteration of the inferior fornices. In the late stages extensive conjunctival scarring, symblepharon formation and entropion may occur. The cornea becomes involved secondarily and may become totally opacified. Less commonly the onset is acute with oedema of the lids, conjunctival ulceration and rapid development of scarring.
Immunofluorescent studies have shown deposition of immunoglobulins (IgG, IgM and IgA) and complement in basement membranes of involved mucosal epithelium including conjunctiva.

Question 89

This patient presented with sudden loss of vision in his fellow eye.

What is the likely cause for the reduced vision in that eye?

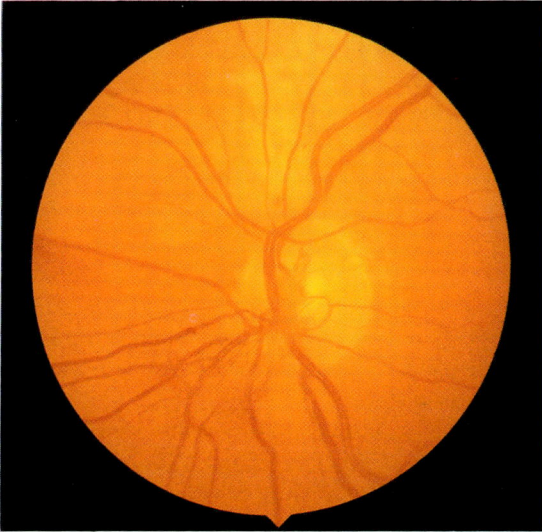

Answer to question 89

Vitreous haemorrhage or a traction retinal detachment involving the macula.

This slide shows a patient with proliferative diabetic retinopathy, a condition which affects about 5% of the diabetic population. It usually develops in patients with preproliferative changes which indicate significant retinal ischaemia and include cotton wool spots, venous dilatation (beading, looping or segmentation), arteriolar narrowing and large blot haemorrhages. New vessels may proliferate on the disc (as in this case) or peripherally, usually along the temporal vascular arcades. Neovascularisation may be complicated by vitreous haemorrhage and formation of fibrous tissue which eventually contracts causing detachment of the retina. Untreated proliferative retinopathy carries a poor prognosis with 70–80% of patients with optic disc neovascularisation progressing to total blindness within five years; peripheral neovascularisation carries a better prognosis.

All patients with proliferative retinopathy require treatment by panretinal photocoagulation where 1000–3000 laser burns are applied to the equatorial and peripheral retina. Following successful treatment regression of new vessels occurs and several trials have shown that such photocoagulation significantly reduces the risk of visual loss.

Question 90

1. What abnormality is shown?
2. What is the diagnosis?
3. List three tests to confirm the diagnosis.

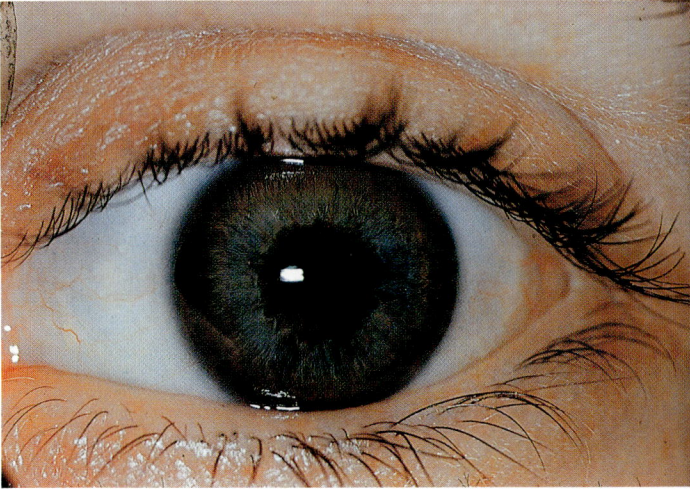

Answer to question 90

1. Kayser—Fleischer ring.
2. Wilson's disease.
3. (a) Low serum ceruloplasmin level.
   (b) Elevated urinary copper excretion.
   (c) Liver biopsy which shows a high copper content.

Wilson's disease is a rare condition caused by a deficiency of the alpha-2-globulin ceruloplasmin. It is characterised by widespread deposition of copper in the tissues, notably in the basal ganglia, liver and kidneys. The Kayser—Fleischer ring which is present in nearly all cases is due to deposition of copper in Descemet's membrane. The green 'sunflower' cataract resulting from copper deposition in the lens is much less common.

Patients may present in infancy with a flapping tremor of the wrists and shoulders and normal liver function or during childhood with hepatosplenomegaly, jaundice and progressive cerebral involvement. The latter manifests as spasticity, dysphagia and dysarthria with or without mental deterioration and emotional instability. Alternatively, cirrhosis may develop without signs of central nervous system involvement. Early treatment with penicillamine can control the disease and render the individual normal mentally and physically. Without treatment this disease is usually fatal within 5–14 years of onset.

Question 91

A 16-year-old girl was referred by her general practitioner because of headaches.

1. What abnormality is shown?
2. What is the treatment?

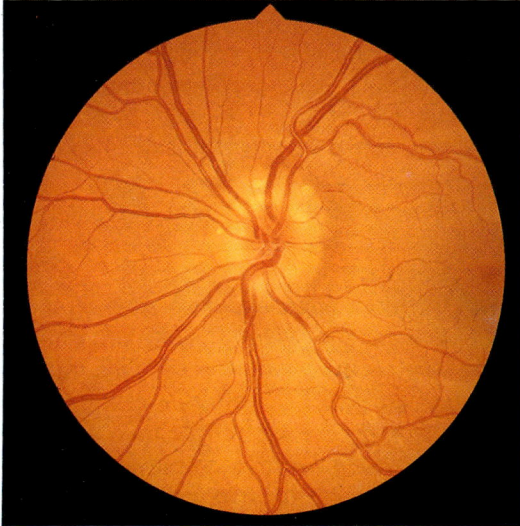

Answer to question 91

1. Optic disc drüsen.
2. No treatment is necessary.

Optic disc drüsen may be confused with papilloedema. The nature of the lesions is unknown, but in many cases they are inherited as an autosomal dominant trait with variable penetrance. In childhood they are 'buried' within the disc and become apparent in adult life.

Clinical features which help distinguish this condition from papilloedema are:

(a) The central disc cup is usually absent and vessels arise from the central apex of the disc.

(b) Anomalous branching and tortuosity of retinal vessels with increased number of major disc vessels.

(c) Peripapillary pigment epithelial atrophy.

(d) Absence of haemorrhages, exudates and cotton wool spots.

(e) Spontaneous venous pulsation may be present.

Disc drüsen may become symptomatic as a result of field loss in the form of arcuate field defects, most commonly inferonasal arcuate field defects, but enlargement of the blind spot and generalised field constriction may occur. Episodes of transient obscuration of vision similar to those seen with raised intracranial pressure are rare and spontaneous haemorrhage on the disc and subretinal peripapillary haemorrhages may occur.

The diagnosis may be confirmed by observing autofluorescence of the drusen or by high-resolution CT scanning, which may show the characteristic small, well-defined areas of high attenuation. Examination of the optic discs of parents and siblings can also be helpful in difficult cases.

Question 92

1. What abnormality is shown?
2. What type of visual field defect is most commonly found in association with this lesion?
3. Which arterial territory is affected?

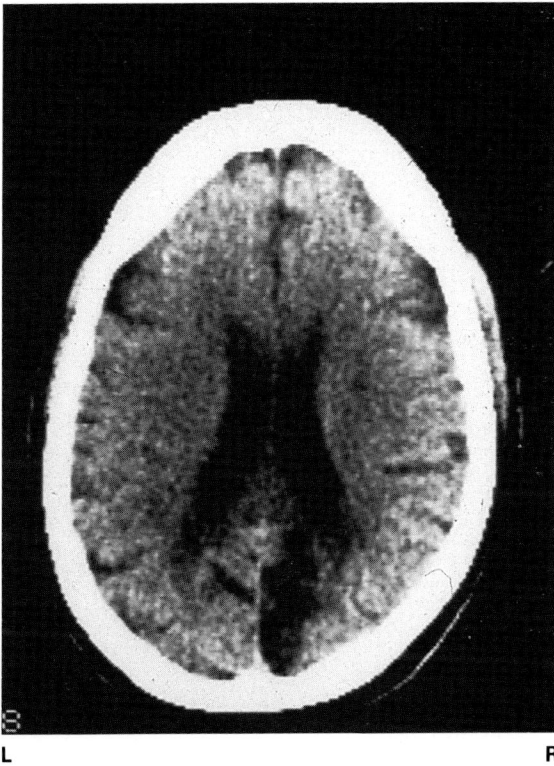

L   R

Answer to question 92

1. Right occipital lobe infarction.
2. Left homonymous hemianopia with macular sparing.
3. Posterior cerebral artery.

Occipital lobe infarction is the commonest cause of an isolated homonymous hemianopia (i.e. without other neurological abnormalities). The phenomenon of macular sparing is diagnostic of such a lesion and is explained by the presence of a collateral circulation to the occipital pole from the middle cerebral artery. Common causes include: hypertension, diabetes mellitus and embolic phenomena arising from the heart or vertebral arteries.

Question 93

This baby developed sticky eyes 10 days after birth.

1. What is the diagnosis?
2. What is the most likely cause?

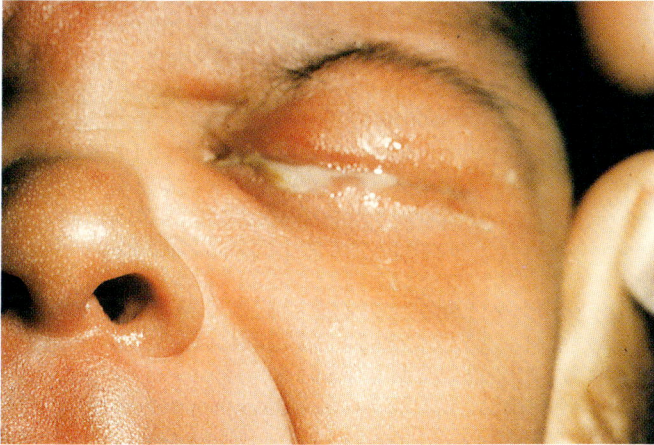

Answer to question 93

1. Ophthalmia neonatorum.
2. *Chlamydia trachomatis.*

Ophthalmia neonatorum is conjunctival inflammation occurring in the first month of life. It is nearly always the result of an infection acquired via the birth canal and in all cases swabs should be obtained in order to identify the infecting organism. The most common cause is now *Chlamydia trachomatis*, which has an incubation period of 5–15 days and presents as an acute mucopurulent conjunctivitis. These cases should be treated with topical tetracycline and because of the associated systemic problems, e.g. pneumonia, systemic erythromycin should also be given. Bacterial conjunctivitis is usually caused by Gram-positive organisms. Gonococcal conjunctivitis is now a rare but potentially blinding cause which may progress rapidly to corneal ulceration and perforation and should be treated aggressively with topical and systemic penicillin. Herpes simplex blepharoconjunctivitis may also present as ophthalmia neonatorum. In all cases the mother and her sexual contacts need to be examined and treated appropriately.

Question 94

This patient complained of drooping of the eyelid.

Name two important associated clinical signs which may provide a clue to the aetiology.

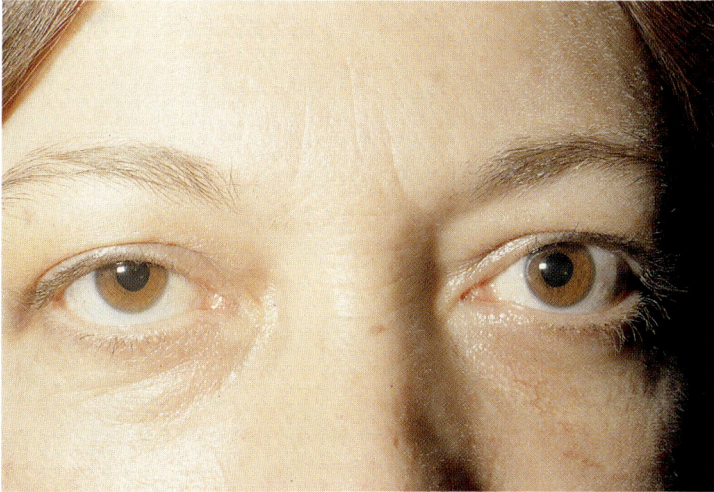

Answer to question 94

The following physical signs should be specifically looked for in patients with ptosis:
(a) Pupillary abnormalities, e.g. miosis in Horner's syndrome, mydriasis in III nerve palsy.
(b) Abnormalities of extraocular movement, e.g. myasthenia gravis, III nerve palsy, ocular myopathies.
(c) Myasthenic signs, e.g. fatigueability, Cogan's lid twitch.
(d) Aberrant eyelid movements, e.g. jaw winking, aberrant III nerve regeneration.

The common causes of ptosis can be classified as follows:

Neurogenic
III nerve palsy.
Horner's syndrome.
Synkinetic: Marcus Gunn jaw winking.
aberrant regeneration of III nerve.

Myogenic
Congenital: simple dystrophy of levator palpebrae superioris.
Acquired: myasthenia gravis.
dystrophia myotonica.
ocular myopathies.

Aponeurotic defects
Senile.

Mechanical
Eyelid tumours.
Dermatochalasis (excessive skin).
Trauma.
Scarring of lid or conjunctiva.

Question 95

This patient who lost central vision in the left eye three years ago presented with distortion of vision in her right eye.

1. What is the diagnosis?
2. What investigation should be performed?

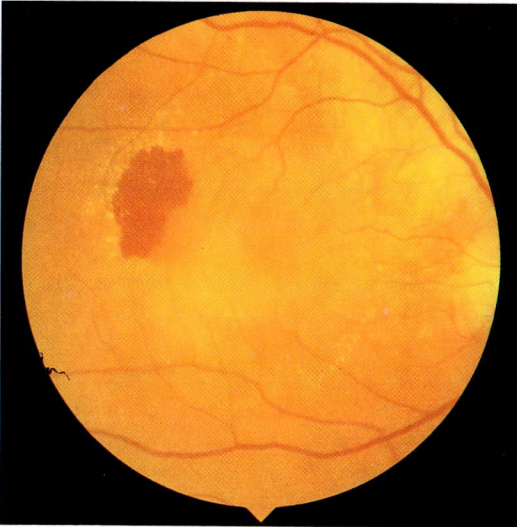

RIGHT EYE

Answer to question 95

1. Disciform degeneration of the macula.
2. Fundus fluorescein angiography.

Senile macular degeneration is the commonest cause of blindness in the elderly population. The disease is bilateral with a 12% incidence of involvement of the second eye each year. Degenerative changes occur in Bruch's membrane and fibrovascular tissue from the choroid passes through defects in the membrane into the subretinal space. In the acute stages this leads to serous elevation of the retina and symptoms of distortion or blurring of vision. At this stage the neovascular complex may be treated with laser therapy, depending on its proximity to the fovea, but must first be accurately located by fundus fluorescein angiography. Untreated, central visual loss occurs from chronic serous detachment of the fovea or subretinal haemorrhage which eventually progresses to a fibrous disciform scar with permanent impairment of central vision. Even in patients who have been successfully treated recurrent disciform lesions may occur and patients should be instructed to attend an ophthalmic unit as soon as they notice any distortion of vision.

Question 96

This 70-year-old man complains of diplopia on looking to the right.

1. What abnormality is shown?
2. What is the differential diagnosis?

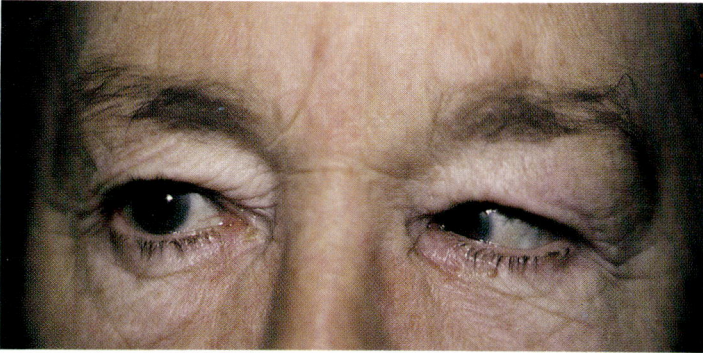

Answer to question 96

1. Reduced abduction of the right eye.
2. (a) Right sixth nerve palsy.
   (b) Myasthenia gravis.
   (c) Thyroid eye disease.
   (d) Medial wall blow-out fracture.
   (e) Other causes: Duane's syndrome, orbital myositis, convergence spasm.

Although a sixth nerve palsy is the commonest cause of an abduction deficit with diplopia, other causes must be considered. Microvascular disease (diabetes mellitus and hypertension) is the commonest cause of an isolated sixth nerve palsy in the elderly and spontaneous recovery within 2–3 months is the rule. In patients with other neurological signs or in whom recovery does not occur full investigation is mandatory.

Question 97

A 32-year-old electrician had experienced several episodes of déjà vu in the previous three months. Neurological examination and EEG were normal and the results of Goldmann perimetry are shown.

1. Which part of the visual pathway is involved and at what site is it involved?
2. What is the blood supply to the involved area?
3. What is the most likely cause of such an isolated field defect?

Right eye

Left eye

Answer to question 97

1. The left optic radiation in the temporal lobe.
2. Middle and posterior cerebral arteries.
3. Cerebral tumours.

Lesions of the optic radiation are common as its lower fibres sweep forwards and downwards into the temporal lobe around the temporal horn of the lateral ventricle (Meyer's loop). Field defects in the temporal lobe often have sloping margins as they are most commonly the result of tumours, whereas vascular lesions, which tend to cause dense field defects with sharply demarcated borders, rarely cause isolated field defects in the temporal lobe but are usually associated with hemiplegia and, if the dominant hemisphere is involved, aphasia.

Question 98

1. What is the diagnosis?
2. What are the typical early visual field defects associated with this condition?

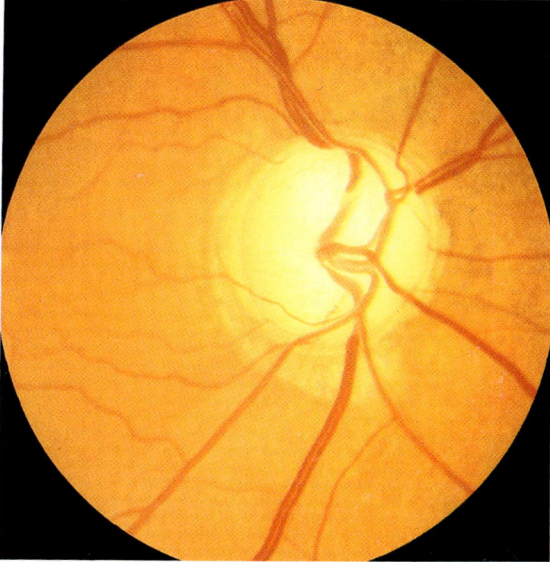

Answer to question 98

1. Glaucomatous optic disc cupping.
2. (a) Generalised peripheral constriction.
   (b) Paracentral nasal scotomas.
   (c) Arcuate field defects.
   (d) Nasal step.

This patient has chronic open-angle glaucoma, i.e. raised intraocular pressures in the presence of optic disc cupping and visual field defects (in the presence of an open anterior chamber angle). These patients are usually asymptomatic until extensive visual field loss has occurred and are often diagnosed on routine examination. Changes at the optic disc suggestive of glaucoma include asymmetry of the cup size between the two eyes, vertical elongation of the optic cup with a cup:disc ratio of more than 0.6, notching and pallor of the neuroretinal rim, nasal displacement of the blood vessels and splinter haemorrhages on the neuroretinal rim.

Question 99

What is the diagnosis?

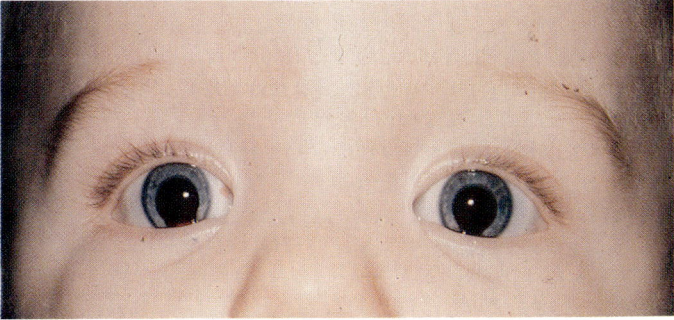

Answer to question 99

Bilateral coloboma of the iris.

Colobomas are congenital abnormalities caused by failure of fusion of the optic cup early in the development of the eye. The defects usually lie inferonasally and may affect the iris, lens, retina, choroid, or optic disc. Colobomas are commonly bilateral, and although most cases are sporadic some are inherited in an autosomal dominant pattern. When the optic disc or retina is involved there may be reduced visual acuity and a visual field defect.

Question 100

A 58-year-old man presented with sudden onset of vertical diplopia, headache and difficulty in walking. On examination he had a vertical deviation of the eyes, coarse rotary nystagmus on left gaze and cerebellar signs on the left side.

What is the likely diagnosis?

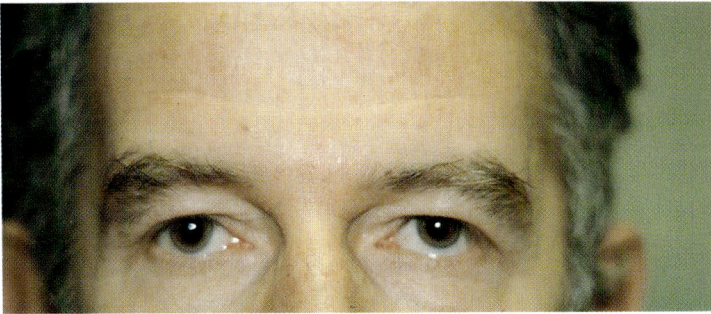

Answer to question 100

Skew deviation.

Skew deviation refers to a vertical misalignment of the eyes secondary to acquired supranuclear or vestibulo-ocular disease. It is usually the result of brainstem ischaemia or posterior fossa haemorrhage. The hypertropia may be the same in all positions of gaze (concomitant) or vary, and the lower eye is more commonly on the side of the brainstem lesion (as in this patient with a right hypotropia and right-sided cerebellar signs). Unilateral internuclear ophthalmoplegia may be associated with skew deviation, usually a unilateral hypertropia.

Skew deviation can be difficult to differentiate from other causes of a vertical deviation, e.g. IV nerve palsy, myasthenia gravis, thyroid eye disease, and in such cases other evidence of neurological disease must be looked for.

Index

Abetalipoproteinaemia, 168
Accommodation loss, 54
Acetylcholine receptor antibodies, 42
Acne rosacea, 155
Acquired immunodeficiency syndrome (AIDS), 56
Acropachy, thyroid, 116
Adenoma sebaceum, 2
Albinism, 101
Amaurosis fugax, 68
Amblyopia
  capillary haemangioma, 112
  strabismic, 83
Angioedema, 29
Angioid streaks, 50, 72, 127
Aniridia, 57
Anisometropia, 83, 112
Ankylosing spondylitis, 110
Anterior ischaemic optic neuropathy, 133
Anterior uveitis, 14
Aorta
  cystic medial necrosis, 22
  dissection, 22
Apraxia, oculomotor, 170
Arcus senilis, 113
Argyll Robertson pupils, 144
Arterial embolism, 184
Arteriogram, cerebral, 157
Arteriovenous malformation, retinal, 9
Arteriovenous nipping, 19
Arthritis, knee, 32
Astrocytoma, retinal, 1
Axillary freckles, 107

Band keratopathy, 14, 165
Basal cell carcinoma, eyelid, 27
Basal skull fracture, 88
Behcet's disease, 31, 110, 152
Bell's palsy, 88
Bell's phenomenon, 87
Benign intracranial hypertension, 77
Bielschowsky head tilt test, 174
Biliary cirrhosis, primary, 90
Bitemporal hemianopia, 70, 149

Blepharitis, 61
  in acne rosacea, 156
Blepharospasm, 47
Blood dyscrasias, 152
Blow-out fracture
  diplopia, 74
  medial wall, 192
Bone, fragility, 24
Bournville's disease, 1
Brainstem lesions, 64, 88
Brushfield spots, 61
Bull's-eye maculopathy, chloroquine-induced, 97
Buphthalmos, 18

C1 esterase inhibitors, reduced levels, 30
Café au lait spots, 107
Candidosis, 56
Capillary haemangioma, 111
Cardiac valve lesions, 24
Caroticocavernous fistula, 96, 135
Carotid artery, DSA, 85
Cataract, 61
  aniridia, 58
  associated systemic disorders, 126
  congenital, 148
  dystrophia myotonica, 142
  green 'sunflower', 180
Central retinal vasculitis, 152
Central retinal vein occlusion (CRVO), 82, 151
Cerebello-pontine angle tumour, 88
Cerebral infarction, 64
Cerebral tumours, 193
Ceruloplasmin deficiency, 180
Cervical cord lesions, 64
Cervical surgical damage, 64
Chlamydia trachomatis, 186
Chloramphenicol, contact dermatitis, 11
Chloroquine, bull's-eye maculopathy induction, 97
Cholesteatoma, 88
Cholesterol emboli, 67
Chorioretinitis, 5
Choroidal haemangioma, 18

Chronic progressive external ophthalmoplegia (CPEO), 59
Clinoid processes, erosion, 15
Coats' disease, 148
Colic, recurrent, 30
Collagen, abnormal synthesis, 24
Collier's sign, 52
Coloboma
of iris, 197
retinal, 148
Compressive optic neuropathy, 37
Congenital Horner's syndrome, 153
Conjunctival inflammation, 3
Conjunctival/episcleral vessels, dilatation, 18
Conjunctivitis, follicular, 26
Contact dermatitis, 11
Convergence retraction nystagmus, 52
Convergence spasm, 192
Corneal pannus, 58
Corneal verticillata, 93
Cotton wool spots, 19, 56
CPEO, 59
Cranial nerve palsies, 42, 56
Craniopharyngioma, 69
Crohn's disease, 110, 144
Cryptococcal retinitis, 56
CT scan
orbital, 95
pituitary fossa, 15
Cytomegalovirus retinitis, 55

Deep tendon reflexes, depressed, 160
Dendritic ulcer, herpetic, 162
Dentinogenesis imperfecta, 24
Dermoid cysts, 96, 103
Diabetes insipidus, 70
Diabetes mellitus, 88, 90, 184
Diabetic retinopathy (maculopathy), 43, 54, 177
proliferative, 82
Digital subtraction angiography (DSA), 85
Diplopia, 158
blow-out fracture, 74
right fourth nerve palsy, 173
Disciform degeneration, macular, 189
Dorsal midbrain syndrome, 51
Drüsen, optic disc, 181

Duane's retraction syndrome, 169, 192
Dysthyroid eye disease, 79, 115
Dystrophia myotonica, 141

Ehlers-Danlos syndrome, 128
Enophthalmos, 63, 74
Epilepsy, 2
focal, 18
Epiloia, 1
Episcleritis, 130, 145
Erythema multiforme, 3, 32
drug-related, 3
Erythema nodosum, 14
Esotropia, infantile, 84
ESR, giant cell arteritis, 46
Eyelid
basal cell carcinoma, 27
plexiform neuroma, 108
retraction, 115
squamous cell carcinoma, 28
xanthelasma, 89

Fabry's disease, 94
Fibromas, subungual, 2
Fluorescein angiography, of fundus, 190
Foreign bodies, 148
Fourth nerve palsy, 173
Fuchs' heterochromic cyclitis, 154

Gaze palsy, 42
Giant cell arteritis, 45
Glaucoma, 22
aniridia, 58
congenital, 18, 108
end-stage, 5
open-angle, chronic, 195
optic disc cupping, 195
Gliomas, optic nerve, 108
Goldmann perimetry, 193
Gonococcal conjunctivitis, 186
Granulomas
sarcoid, 14
Wernicke's, 96, 144, 172
Graves' ophthalmopathy, 79, 115
Guillain-Barré syndrome, 88

Haemangioma, racemose, retinal, 9
Haemophilus influenzae, 36
Headache, ipsilateral, 158
Hemianopia, 70

Hemifacial spasm, 131
Hemisensory deficit, 18
Herpes simplex, 3, 161
  blepharoconjunctivitis, 186
Herpes zoster, 88
  ophthalmicus, 56, 123
Heterochromia, iris, 18
Heterochromic cyclitis of Fuchs, 154
Hilar lymphadenopathy, 14
HLA-B5, Behçet's disease, 32
HLA-DW5, iritis, 130
Hollenhorst plaques, 67
Holmes-Adie pupil, 159
Homocystinuria, 22
Homonymous hemianopia, 70, 184
Horner's syndrome, 64, 145
  congenital, 153
Hydrocephalus, 70
Hypercalcaemia, 166
Hyperlipidaemia, 90
Hyperparathyroidism, 166
Hypertension, 88, 184
  intracranial benign, 77
Hypertensive retinopathy, 19, 54
  grades, 20
Hypertropia, 200
Hypogonadism, 100
Hypopituitarism, 69
Hysteria, 6

Immunoglobulin deposition,
  conjunctival, 176
Infraorbital nerve contusion, 73
Internuclear ophthalmoplegia, 33,
  42, 200
Intracranial hypertension, benign,
  77
Iridocyclitis, juvenile rheumatoid
  arthritis, 130
Iris
  atrophy, 154
  heterochromia, 18
  nodules, 61
  pigmentation disorders, 64
Iritis
  acute, 109
  Behçet's disease, 32
  posterior synechiae, 145

Jacksonian epilepsy, 18
Joints, hypermobility, 24
Jugular foramen, tumours, 64

Kaposi's sarcoma, 56
Kayser-Fleischer ring, 179
Kearns Sayre syndrome, 60
Keratic precipitates (mutton fat), 13
Keratitis, in acne rosacea, 156
Keratoconjunctivitis sicca, 130
Keratoconus, 61
Keratopathy, band, 14, 165
Korsakoff's psychosis, 66

Laurence-Moon-Biedl syndrome, 99
Lens, upward subluxation, 22
Leucocoria (white pupil), 147
Levator palpebrae superioris,
  paralysis, 54
Lisch nodules, 108
Lower motor neurone lesion, 87
Lupus erythematosus, systemic
  (SLE), 144

Macular degeneration, senile, 189
Macular hypoplasia, 58
Macular star, 19
Marcus Gunn jaw winking ptosis,
  137
Marfan's syndrome, 21
Medial longitudinal fasciculus
  (MLF) lesions, 34
Meibomian gland carcinoma, 28
Meige's syndrome, 48
Melanoma
  iris, 154
  malignant, eyelid, 28
Melkersson's syndrome, 88
Meningioma, 164
Meningoencephalitis, 32
Mental retardation, 2, 18, 100
Methylcholine hypersensitivity, 160
Microaneurysms, diabetic, 43
Middle cerebral artery, 193
Middle ear disease, 88
Miosis, 63
  bilateral, 145
Moebius' syndrome, 169
Molluscum contagiosum, 25
Mucous membrane pemphigoid,
  benign, 175
Multiple myeloma, 152
Multiple periventricular lucencies,
  7
Multiple sclerosis (MS), 34, 88
  MRI, 7

Myasthenia gravis, 34, 41, 192
tests, 42
Myasthenia, ocular, 42
Mycoplasma pneumoniae, 3
Myelinated nerve fibres, 119
Myopia, 22, 61
Myxoedema, 90
pretibial, 116

Nephroblastoma (Wilms' tumour),
58
Neurofibromatosis, 108
Neurosarcoidosis, 14
Non-accidental injury, 139
Nystagmus, 34
aniridia, 58
Nystagmus blockage syndrome,
170

Obesity, truncal, 100
Occipital lobe infarction, 5, 183
Oculomotor apraxia, 170
Ophthalmia neonatorum, 185
Ophthalmoplegia
chronic progressive external
(CPEO), 59
external, 142
internuclear, 33, 42, 200
Optic disc drüsen, 181
Optic nerve, hypoplasia, 58
Optic nerve compression, 50
Optic nerve lesions, 37
Optic nerve myelination, 119
Optic neuritis, 7, 91
Optic neuropathy, anterior
ischaemic, 133
Orbit
blow-out fracture, 73
tumours, 95
Orbital cellulitis, 35
Orbital myositis, 192
Orbital pseudotumour, 96
Orbital varices, 96
Osteogenesis imperfecta, 23
Otosclerosis, 24

Paget's disease of bone, 49, 128
Pancoast's syndrome, 64
Papilloedema
AIDS, 56
chronic, 5
drüsen differentiation, 182

Parinaud's syndrome, 51
Pemphigoid, ocular cicatricial, 175
Periphlebitis
focal, 14
retinal, 152
Periventricular lucencies, multiple,
7
Phakomatosis, 108
Phospholipid/cholesterol
deposition, corneal, 113
Pigmentary retinopathy, 142
Pilocarpine hypersensitivity, 160
Pineal tumour, MRI, 51
Pituitary fossa, enlargement, 15
Pituitary tumour, 15, 150
Polyarteritis nodosa, 144
Polycythaemia rubra vera, 152
Polymyalgia rheumatica, 46
Port wine naevus, 17
Posterior cerebral artery, 193
Posterior cerebral artery infarction,
184
Posterior communicating artery
aneurysm, 54, 157, 164
Posterior synechiae, iritis, 145
Posterior uveitis, 14
Pregnancy, lower motor neurone
lesion, 88
Prematurity retinopathy, 82, 148
Preseptal cellulitis, 36
Pretibial myxoedema, 116
Primary biliary cirrhosis, 90
Progressive external
ophthalmoplegia, chronic
(CPEO), 59
Proliferative diabetic retinopathy,
82
Proptosis, 95
Pseudo Argyll Robertson pupils,
145
Pseudo Foster-Kennedy syndrome,
134
Pseudotumour cerebri, 77
Pseudoxanthoma elasticum, 71, 128
Psoriatic arthritis, 110
Pterygium, 75
Ptosis, 63
causes/physical signs, 187
dystrophia myotonica, 142
Marcus Gunn, 137
Pupil, dilatation, 54
Pupillary light-near dissociation, 52

Racemose haemangioma, retinal, 9
Red eye, 117
Reduced abduction, 191
Refsum's disease, 168
Reiter's syndrome, 110
Respiratory tract, oedema, 30
Retina, haemorrhages, 19
Retinal detachment, 22, 82
    traction, 177
Retinal dysplasias, 148
Retinal exudation, 32
Retinal oedema, 32
Retinal phakoma, 1
Retinitis pigmentosa, 5, 99, 167
    sectoral, 168
Retinoblastoma, 148
Retinochondritis, toxoplasmosis,
    105
Retinopathy
    hypertensive, 19
    prematurity, 82, 148
    sickle cell, 82
Retrobulbar neuritis, 92
Rheumatoid arthritis, 122, 129, 144
Rhinophyma, 156
Rubeosis iridis, 82

Saccades
    slow, 34
    upgaze paresis, 52
Sarcoidosis, 13, 88, 152
Scleritis, 130, 144
Scleromalacia perforans, 121, 130
Scotoma
    left central, 91
    retinitis pigmentosa, 168
Senile macular degeneration, 189
Sickle cell anaemia, 128
Sickle cell retinopathy, 82
Siderosis, ocular, 154
Sixth nerve palsy, 192
Skew deviation, 199
Skull, tramline calcification, 18
Spheno-orbital encephalocele, 108
Sphenoid wing meningioma, 39
Squint, 61
    postoperative conditions, 34
    right convergent, 83
Staphylococcus aureus, 36
Stevens-Johnson syndrome, 3
Strabismic amblyopia, 83
Strabismus fixus, 170

Strawberry naevus, 111
Streptococcus pneumoniae, 36
Streptococcus pyogenes, 36
Sturge-Weber syndrome, 17
Supraorbital pain, 158
Symblepharon, 4
Systemic lupus erythematosus
    (SLE), 144

Temporal lobe, left optic radiation
    lesion, 193
Tensilon test, 42
Third cranial nerve
    aberrant regeneration, 163
    palsy, 53
    trauma, 164
Thrombophlebitis, 32
Thyroid acropachy, 116
Thyroid eye disease, 34, 95, 192
Thyrotoxicosis, 42
Toxocara endophthalmitis, 148
Toxoplasma gondii, 106
Toxoplasmosis, 56
    retinochondritis, 105
Traction retinal detachment, 177
Trisomy 21, 62
Tuberculum sellae meningioma, 37
Tuberous sclerosis, 1
    cutaneous lesions, 2
Tubers, retinal, 1

Ulcerative colitis, 110
Uniocular visual loss, transient, 68
Urticarial whealing, 30
Uveitis
    acute anterior, 109
    Behçet's disease, 32
    sarcoid-associated, 13

Vasculitis, retinal, 14, 56
Venous stasis retinopathy, 152
Verticillata, corneal, 93
Vesicopapular eruptions, 32
Visual field defects, AIDS, 56
Vitreous, persistent primary
    hyperplastic, 148
Vitreous haemorrhage, 177
Von Recklinghausen's disease, 108

Waldenström's
    macroglobulinaemia, 152

Wegener's granulomatosis, 96, 144, 172
Wernicke's encephalopathy, 65
White pupil (leucocoria), 147
Wilms' tumour, 58

Wilson's disease, 180
Xanthelasma, eyelid, 89
Xerostomia, 130